IMPORTANT NOTICE
This book is intended not as a substitute for personal
medical advice but as a supplement to that advice for
the patient who wishes to understand more about his
or her condition.

Before taking any form of treatment
YOU SHOULD ALWAYS CONSULT YOUR MEDICAL
PRACTITIONER

In particular (without limit) you should note that
advances in medical science occur rapidly and some of
the information about drugs and treatment contained in
this booklet may very soon be out of date.

Editorial consultants: Miss Monica McGill and Mr Matthew Barber

Acknowledgements
To my patients who have and continue to inspire me, I thank you all. Thanks
also to Kirsty Birrell who is such an enormous help to me in looking after my
many patients. I am grateful for the assistance of Carol Lindays and Mandy
Stewart in locating suitable mammograms for inclusion in this book.
Support as always has been forthcoming from my wife Pam and sons Oliver
and Jonathan, who continue to tolerate the hours that I spend writing books
like this. Thanks also to Jan Mauritzen for juggling my diary and ensuring that I
occasionally achieve something in my life. Last, but not least, enormous thanks
to Monica McGill who has contributed significantly to this book by not only
making sense of my garbled words and scribbles but also improving them and
ensuring that they are understandable.

Family Doctor Publications, PO Box 4664, Poole, Dorset BH15 1NN

ISBN 13: 987-1903-474-62-4
ISBN 10: 1-903474-62-0

7oooooo40201

Contents

About the author

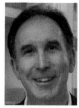

Professor Mike Dixon is a Consultant Surgeon and Professor of Surgery at the Edinburgh Breast Unit. He is Clinical Director of the Breakthrough Research Unit in Edinburgh. He works in the UK's largest breast unit in Edinburgh. As well as having written more than 16 books and more than 250 papers, he has an enormously busy clinical practice in breast disease.

He is acknowledged as one of the leading breast surgeons in the country; he was the inaugural editor of *The Breast* and was on the first editorial board of the *British Medical Journal*. He was also the first section editor for breast disease for *Clinical Evidence*, which is now available for patients.

Professor Dixon is a medical consultant on the information leaflets currently produced on breast cancer by Breast Cancer Care and Macmillan Cancer Relief. Professor Dixon has been an invited speaker at all the major meetings on breast cancer throughout the world and is co-chairman of the annual Miami Breast Cancer Conference.

He originally started work in the NHS as a porter in Sheffield where he worked for 15 months before starting medical school. He also spent two three-month periods as a nursing auxiliary. It is his undoubted expertise combined with his down-to-earth, straightforward approach that makes him the ideal person to answer your questions about breast cancer.

Introduction

How common is breast cancer?

Breast cancer is the most common type of cancer among women. Each year there are approximately 41,000 new cases in the UK and over one million worldwide.

Although breast cancer is much more common in women, it can also affect men and in the UK approximately 300 men every year develop breast cancer. One in nine women will develop breast cancer at some time in her life.

This booklet covers possible causes, screening and symptoms of breast cancer, and how it is diagnosed and treated. It also contains important information to help women cope with the disease.

Much research continues into the causes of breast cancer, as well as new ways to prevent, diagnose and treat it. As a result men and women diagnosed now with breast cancer have a much higher chance of living and surviving it.

How do breasts grow and change?

Breasts start to develop a few weeks after the embryo is formed in the womb. At about six months of pregnancy, some cells grow inwards and these cells develop to form what will be the baby's nipples and milk ducts. By the time the baby is born the basic breast structure is in place.

In most girls, breasts start to develop between the ages of nine and eleven years but this process can begin earlier or later. Even when fully developed, the breasts at this stage are not capable of producing milk. It is also common for boys to get some breast development during puberty. This can be embarrassing but is usually only temporary and in over 80 per cent disappears within a year or two.

During pregnancy a woman's breasts increase in size and approximately double in weight as milk-producing cells multiply and the system of ducts expands. The nipples get darker in colour during pregnancy and the blood vessels under the skin of the breast become more prominent. All these changes take place as a result of the various hormones that are produced during pregnancy and most of these changes are only temporary.

What is a breast made of?
The easiest way to understand how the inside of the breast is arranged is by comparing it with an upturned tree. The leaves of the breast 'tree' are known as lobules. They produce milk, which drains along the branches of the breast tree forming a network of small ducts. These in turn drain into 12 or 15 large ducts, which empty on to the surface of the nipple. The nipple is equivalent to the bush's trunk.

As with a tree, the breast's branching network of ducts is irregular and complicated and not arranged symmetrically into segments as, for example, is found in an orange.

Anatomy of the female breast

The breast can be visualised as an upside-down tree. The leaves of the tree are the lobules and the trunk the nipple.

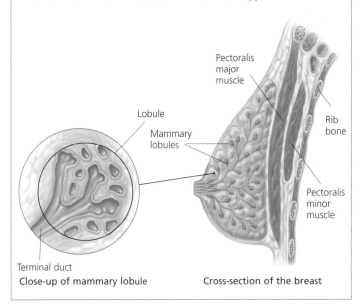

Lobule

Mammary lobules

Pectoralis major muscle

Rib bone

Pectoralis minor muscle

Terminal duct

Close-up of mammary lobule

Cross-section of the breast

The breast also contains blood and lymph vessels. The lymph vessels carry clear fluid called lymph from the breast tissue to lymph nodes close to the breast. The nodes that drain most of the lymph from the breast are in the area under the arm and are called the axillary nodes. A small amount of lymph does drain inward to lymph nodes underneath the breastbone.

Lymph nodes are important in the body's defence systems, and are involved with dealing with bacteria, cancer cells or other harmful substances. Cancer cells that enter lymph channels can pass to draining lymph nodes where some of the cells grow and result in lymph node enlargement.

The space between the branches of the breast tree is made up of fat and this gives the breast a soft feel. Women's breasts are rarely the same size as each other and breasts can feel different at different times of the monthly menstrual cycle, often swelling and becoming tender in the week before a period. As a woman gets older the amount of breast tissue in the breast reduces and is replaced by fat so the breasts become softer.

What is breast cancer?

Many cells in the human body are growing at any one time but their growth is very carefully controlled so that the number of cells produced matches the number of cells that are dying. A cancer develops when cells grow or divide at a faster rate than normal but escape from the normal mechanisms that control cell growth.

This results in the development of a cancerous lump (primary tumour), which if untreated gets bigger and bigger, as the cells continue to divide and so multiply.

Lumps are common in the breast and there are many causes for breast lumps other than breast cancer. Only about one in eight lumps is cancer (malignant growth) and the rest are not serious or life threatening and do not spread to other areas of the body. These are known as benign lumps. The most common treatment for a cancer in the breast is surgery to remove the cancer.

If the lump continues to grow, some of the cells may develop the ability to move away from the lump to other parts of the body, where they grow to form secondary tumours. This is called spread or metastasis of a cancer.

The cancer cells can spread if they enter the lymph channels, through which they travel to other lymph

How a tumour forms

A cancerous tumour begins as a single cell. If it is not destroyed by the body's immune system, it will double into two cells, which in turn divide into four and so on.

Cancerous cell

First doubling

Second doubling

nodes where they can continue to grow and result in enlarged lymph glands which may be felt, for instance, as a lump under the arm.

If cancer is present in the lymph nodes this can be treated by surgery to remove the affected nodes or by radiotherapy, which is effective at destroying cancer cells.

Cells can also get into blood vessels and cells that get into the bloodstream can result in the development of new lumps (metastases) in different areas of the body.

If cancer cells start to grow in an important area such as the lungs, liver or brain, or if cells grow in bones, they can cause a range of different symptoms and problems as they disrupt normal function of that organ.

Treatment for cancer that has spread usually includes some form of drug treatment that treats the cancer wherever it is in the body. Radiotherapy can be combined with the drug treatment to treat areas where the cancer cells are growing.

KEY POINTS

■ Most lumps in the breast are not serious

■ Cancer is the uncontrolled overgrowth of a group of cells

■ Another term for cancer is a malignant tumour

■ Cells from a malignant tumour, if left untreated, may continue to grow and eventually invade and spread to damage other tissues

■ As a cancer grows, some cancer cells may break away from the cancer and enter the bloodstream or the lymphatic system; this results in cancer cells spreading from the original cancer (the primary tumour) to form new cancers or secondary tumours in other organs – called metastases

■ Cancer cells that get into the lymphatic system can sometimes be felt as lumps under the arm in the lymph glands

■ Even if a cancer has spread, it can be treated

Who develops breast cancer?

How likely am I to get breast cancer?

No one knows why some people develop breast cancer and others do not. What is clear is that injuries such as bumping, bruising or touching the breast do not cause cancer. It is also not possible to catch cancer from a person who has it.

Many factors play a part in determining who develops breast cancer and it is not simple to try to work out any individual's personal level of risk. Most women have little or no control over most of the important risk factors for breast cancer. Research has shown that certain risk factors make it more likely that some women will develop breast cancer than others.

A risk factor is something that increases a person's chance of developing a disease. Experts have identified the factors that seem to make it more likely that a woman will develop breast cancer. However, even if you have lots of risk factors you will not necessarily get breast cancer and, even if you have no risk factors, you may still be unfortunate enough to develop it.

Risk factors
Female sex
Being female is a definite risk factor for developing breast cancer because over 99 per cent of all breast cancers develop in women. Breast cancer in men is very rare and fewer than 1 in 200 of all breast cancers develops in men. There are about 300 new breast cancers in men per year in the UK compared with 41,000 in women.

Age
Breast cancer risk increases as you get older. Older women are at the greatest risk – breast cancer is uncommon under the age of 40 years. More than 80 per cent of all breast cancers develop in women over the age of 50 and 40 per cent of women with breast cancer are aged 70 or older.

An estimate of the risk of developing breast cancer by age

Age group	No. of women who get breast cancer up to this age
To age 25	1 in 15,000 women
To age 30	1 in 1,900 women
To age 40	1 in 200 women
To age 50	1 in 50 women
To age 60	1 in 23 women
To age 70	1 in 15 women
To age 80	1 in 11 women
To age 85	1 in 10 women
Lifetime risk (all ages)	1 in 9 women

Family history

Fewer than one in ten (ten per cent) women who develop breast cancer do so because they have inherited some kind of genetic abnormality that makes them more susceptible to develop this condition.

Women with inherited risk

Everyone has two copies of every gene – you inherit one copy of each gene from your mother and one from your father. Even if your mother has had breast cancer and is carrying an abnormal gene only one of the two copies of the gene is abnormal and the other copy works normally.

That means that every child of a mother with an abnormal gene has a 50% (1 in 2) chance of inheriting the normal gene and a 50% (1 in 2) chance of inheriting the abnormal gene.

So even if your mother is carrying a genetic abnormality there is no certainty that you will have it.

Women who are at increased risk of breast cancer because there is likely to be an abnormal gene running in their family are identified because:

- There are several members in the family who have had breast cancer

- Relatives have developed breast cancer while under the age of 50 years; the earlier in life this happens, the greater the risk that cancer has developed because of an inherited abnormality

- Relatives have had cancer affecting both breasts or relatives have had certain other cancers while young, particularly cancer of the ovaries (in women), and colon and prostate (in men).

There are various ways of identifying women with this kind of risk and these are given in the boxes. In a small number of women it is possible to perform a gene test to identify if they have an abnormal gene that makes them more likely to develop a breast cancer.

Familial breast cancer

Criteria for identifying women at substantial increased risk

The following categories identify women who have three or more times the population risk of developing breast cancer and who would benefit from regular screening from a young age. A woman who has:

- one first-degree relative with bilateral breast cancer or breast and ovarian cancer **or**

- one first-degree relative with breast cancer diagnosed under the age of 40 years or one first-degree male relative with breast cancer diagnosed at any age **or**

- two first- or second-degree relatives with breast cancer diagnosed under the age of 60 years or ovarian cancer at any age on the same side of the family **or**

- three first- or second-degree relatives with breast and ovarian cancer on the same side of the family.

A first-degree female relative is a mother, sister or daughter.
A first-degree male relative is a father, brother or son.
A second-degree female relative is a grandmother, granddaughter, aunt or niece.

Familial breast cancer (contd)

Criteria for identifying women at very high risk in whom gene testing may be appropriate

- Families with four or more relatives affected with either breast or ovarian cancer in three generations and one alive affected individual.

There is a network of family history clinics throughout the UK who look after women identified on the basis of their family history as being at increased risk.

They offer breast screening, starting at a much younger age than the general population screening which starts at age 50. Screening is not only by mammography but in known gene carriers may include magnetic resonance imaging (MRI) performed every year.

These family history clinics have access to genetic testing and can refer women to hospital for consideration of surgery if considered appropriate for women carrying a faulty breast cancer gene.

Previous treatment for breast cancer

Women who develop cancer in one breast are more likely than the general population to develop a cancer in their other breast. Each year between 4 and 6 of every 1,000 women who have a cancer in one breast will develop cancer in their opposite breast.

It is for this reason that such women should have lifelong breast screening with regular breast X-rays (mammograms). Hormonal drugs that are used to treat breast cancer reduce the risk of developing another breast cancer by about 50 per cent.

Benign breast conditions

Most types of benign (non-cancerous) breast problems
do not significantly increase the risk of developing
breast cancer. This includes cysts and common lumps
in younger women (fibroadenomas).

Some women who have had a non-cancerous
condition where there is an overgrowth (hyperplasia) of
their breast cells which are different from normal cells
(atypical), called atypical hyperplasia, are at increased
risk of developing breast cancer.

This condition is usually diagnosed after biopsy of a
lump or removal of an area of abnormality found on a
mammogram during breast screening. Women with
this condition need regular check-ups.

Reproductive and menstrual history

The older a woman is when she has her first child the
greater her chance of developing breast cancer. Having
children while young (under 20) protects against breast
cancer. A woman having her first child when she is
over the age of 34 years is at a greater risk of
developing breast cancer later in life than a woman
who has never had a child.

Women who have their first menstrual period at an
early age (below the age of 12 years) or go through
the menopause late (after the age of 55 years) are at a
slightly increased risk of developing breast cancer.

Taking the contraceptive pill

There is a very slightly increased risk of a woman
developing breast cancer while she is taking the oral
contraceptive pill. However, as the overall risk of breast
cancer developing in young women is small, the extra
risk associated with taking the pill is exceedingly small

and not clinically important. Any risk associated with pill usage is short-lived and disappears quickly after stopping the pill.

Taking hormone replacement therapy

Women who take hormone replacement therapy (HRT), particularly if they take a combination of oestrogen and progestogen, have an increased chance of developing breast cancer.

The risk of developing breast cancer is greater the longer a woman takes the HRT. The risks associated with the use of oestrogen-only HRT are much less than those associated with combined oestrogen and progestogen preparations.

Although HRT is effective at controlling menopausal symptoms such as hot flushes and night sweats, and protects against osteoporosis (thinning of the bones), there are some concerns that it increases the risk of strokes and blood clots as well as breast cancer.

HRT can be taken to improve menopausal symptoms such as hot flushes, vaginal dryness and loss of concentration, but should be given in the smallest effective dose for the shortest duration (two to three years).

One problem with HRT is that when women stop it menopausal symptoms usually come back. This suggests that you cannot prevent menopausal symptoms with HRT; all you do is postpone these symptoms until you are older.

Tibolone as an alternative to oestrogen with progestogen

Tibolone is an interesting drug that has been used for women to control menopausal symptoms. It is a type of 'HRT' that does not contain oestrogen. It mimics the actions of oestrogen, improving menopausal symptoms and protecting the bones.

However, tibolone can be taken only by women who are truly postmenopausal, that is women who have had no menstrual bleeding for at least a year.

Studies looking at the relationship between tibolone and breast cancer have been conflicting. In theory, tibolone should not increase the risk of breast cancer and it should be much safer than combinations of oestrogen and progestogen. One study has, however, shown an increased risk of breast cancer in women taking tibolone whereas another study did not. At present therefore it is not yet clear whether tibolone does not increase the risk of breast cancer similar to other forms of HRT.

A recent study has shown that, when given to women with breast cancer who have severe menopausal symptoms, tibolone, similar to other forms of HRT, increases the chances of the cancer returning.

Taking HRT long term

Women who want to continue to use HRT long term and have had a hysterectomy can take oestrogen alone because this increases the risk of breast cancer less than combined HRT.

For women who still have their uterus, a combination of oestrogen alone with progestogen delivered locally to the lining of the uterus through a Mirena coil may be a safer option than continuing on combined continuous oestrogen and progestogen for more than two to three years.

How does the risk factor change with HRT use?
There is an extra risk of getting breast cancer with each year of taking HRT. These risks add up, particularly with combined oestrogen and progestogen, amounting to a doubling of risk after five years of use. This risk seems to be independent of the dose of oestrogen used, type of oestrogen and mode of delivery (oral or skin patches). The same is true for progestogen.

It is not clear whether progestogen-only HRT increases the risk of breast cancer. Vaginal oestrogen does not seem to increase the risk.

Is HRT worth the increased risk of breast cancer?
The decision whether to take HRT is an individual one between you and your doctor, based on the pros and cons for each individual woman. There are other options for controlling menopausal symptoms and treating osteoporosis other than taking HRT.

For a fuller discussion of HRT see the Family Doctor Book *Understanding the Menopause & HRT*.

Breast-feeding
Breast-feeding a child results in a slight reduction in the chances of developing breast cancer. The highest benefit is from breast-feeding at a young age and the best protection is in women who breast-feed for long periods of time.

Physical activity
There is some evidence that regular exercise reduces the risk of developing breast cancer. It appears that women gain most benefit if they exercise regularly, three or four times a week, over many years.

Being overweight

Being seriously overweight when you are older (postmenopausal) increases breast cancer risk. You are considered to be overweight if you are more than 1.5 times the average weight for your height.

There is also a link between breast cancer and eating a diet that is high in fat, but no one yet knows how this is connected. There is no evidence that dairy products increase the risk of developing breast cancer or that avoiding dairy products reduces the risk of developing breast cancer.

Ethnicity

Breast cancer occurs more often in white women than in women of Latin, Asian or African origin.

Country of birth

The proportion of women affected by breast cancer varies between different countries. The highest incidence is in women born in North America or northern Europe. There is a lower risk of breast cancer in women who are born in Asia or Africa.

What is interesting is that women born in Asia or Africa who move to America and adopt a western lifestyle, including a western diet, show, over a 20-year period, the same risk of breast cancer as women born in America.

These observations explain why it is believed that the major reasons for women developing breast cancer are environmental, that is related to where women live and what they eat rather than related to inherited risk from faulty genes.

Previous radiotherapy to the chest

Women who have had radiotherapy to the chest, including the breasts, before the age of 30 are at some increased risk of breast cancer. This includes women treated with radiotherapy for Hodgkin's lymphoma.

Studies show that the younger a woman is when she receives radiation treatment, the greater the risk of breast cancer development later in life. Regular screening starting at a young age is available for women with Hodgkin's lymphoma who have been treated with radiotherapy.

Drinking alcohol and smoking

Some studies have shown a link between drinking alcohol and the risk of developing breast cancer. Women who drink alcohol regularly have a higher risk of developing breast cancer than those who drink no alcohol or drink in moderation.

The relationship between smoking and breast cancer is not clear. Overall there does not appear to be any direct evidence that smoking increases the risk of breast cancer, but it does of course increase the risk of many other cancers and also increases the risk of some benign breast conditions, particularly infection in the area behind the nipple.

Some studies have shown that there may be an increased risk of developing breast cancer at a young age in women who smoke. There are also some data showing that women who are exposed to passive smoking, because their partner smokes, are also at a slightly increased risk of developing breast cancer.

Genes that cause breast cancer

Every individual is different. We are all a mix of our parents. Half the genes in our bodies are inherited from our mother and half from our father.

Some individuals inherit an abnormal gene from their mother or father that puts them at increased risk of developing certain diseases. No one yet knows how many genes are associated with an increased risk of breast cancer but five major genes have been identified so far.

- About five per cent of all breast cancers develop in women because they have inherited an abnormal gene from either their mother or their father.

- About one in three of the inherited cases of breast cancer is thought to result from an abnormality in the gene called *BRCA*-1.

- Another third of inherited breast cancers are related to another gene called *BRCA*-2.

- Another three genes and a number of other undiscovered genes are responsible for the remainder.

BRCA-1 and *BRCA*-2 genes

Women who inherit a faulty *BRCA*-1 or *BRCA*-2 gene have an increased lifetime risk not only of breast cancer but also of ovarian and possibly colon (large bowel) cancer.

Men who carry a faulty *BRCA*-2 gene are also at higher risk of developing breast cancer. These men are also at risk of getting prostate cancer.

Testing for faulty *BRCA*-1 and *BRCA*-2 genes is possible but it takes two months to get a result and the testing can fail to detect some individuals with significant gene changes if the test does not check the whole of the gene.

Before women can be offered a test it is necessary to show that someone in their family who has had a breast cancer has an abnormal gene. Women who come from such affected families may then be given the opportunity to find out if they are carrying an abnormal gene and are at increased risk.

Women who are shown on testing to have an abnormal gene have between a 60 per cent and an 85 per cent chance of developing breast cancer at some time in their life. Such women also have a higher risk of developing ovarian cancer.

It is important to realise that if you are carrying a faulty breast cancer gene it does not necessarily mean that you will get breast cancer. This is because everybody has two copies of the same gene, so if one is faulty then, provided that the other one continues to work normally, cancer will not develop. More often than not, however, at some point the other gene stops working and then cancer develops.

In women who carry a faulty *BRCA*-1 or *BRCA*-2 gene the breast cancers that do develop tend to occur at a young age. It is estimated that about 1 in 800 women carries a faulty *BRCA*-1 gene. There is a higher incidence of faulty genes in certain groups of women, for example, Ashkenazi Jewish women have a much higher risk of having a faulty *BRCA*-1 or *BRCA*-2 gene and so not surprisingly they have a much higher incidence of breast and ovarian cancer than other women of a similar age.

p53 gene

Other genes associated with breast cancer include the p53 gene which, if faulty, results in women developing breast cancer early. In these women, breast cancer is often bilateral (affects both breasts).

A faulty p53 gene is responsible for the Li–Fraumeni syndrome. In this syndrome there are usually cases of breast cancer in the family and also a history of tumours of bone often affecting children.

It is thought that the p53 gene is a gene that controls the growth of cells. When it is faulty there is not enough control so cells overgrow and cancer can develop. Although other faulty genes have been identified, they are much less common.

Reducing risk from faulty genes

If a woman is tested and found to be carrying an abnormal gene she may wish to have regular tests to diagnose a cancer early if one develops. This would mean having regular intensive breast screening starting at an early age.

For a woman with a strong family history of breast cancer or where gene tests suggest that she is carrying an abnormal gene, other options are surgery to remove all breast tissue or taking part in prevention studies to try to prevent breast cancer development.

Prevention of breast cancer

Oestrogen is an important factor in breast cancer development. By interfering with the action of oestrogen it should be possible to reduce the number of women who develop breast cancer. Oestrogen works by binding to receptors on the surface of breast cells.

Two groups of drugs have been studied:

1. Drugs such as tamoxifen and raloxifene work by binding to the oestrogen receptor and blocking these receptors, so the oestrogen that the body produces cannot get to the breast cells.

2. Drugs called aromatase inhibitors work by stopping the body producing oestrogen, but these drugs are effective only in women whose ovaries are no longer working, that is postmenopausal women.

Tamoxifen

Tamoxifen can reduce the occurrence of breast cancer by almost a half when given to women at increased risk. But only hormone-sensitive – known as oestrogen receptor-positive – cancers are prevented. There are, however, significant problems with tamoxifen in that it causes unpleasant and sometimes serious side effects.

To date none of the trials has shown that women who took tamoxifen lived longer. Women in the tamoxifen prevention trials who seemed to benefit most included those with atypical hyperplasia (see page 209) and those with a type of change in the breast called lobular carcinoma *in situ* or lobular neoplasia (see page 73).

Despite the success of tamoxifen in reducing the number of women who developed breast cancer, the overall message from the UK tamoxifen study was that the benefits are balanced by the risks. Based on this conclusion tamoxifen is not in routine use as a preventive agent in the UK but can be given to individuals after a detailed discussion of the pros and cons of its benefits and risks.

Newer drugs
Raloxifene

Raloxifene is a tamoxifen-like drug with potentially less serious side effects. In American studies it has been shown to be as effective as tamoxifen at preventing breast cancer.

Raloxifene is not used routinely for breast cancer prevention in the UK. It is, however, used in postmenopausal women to treat osteoporosis under the trade name Evista.

Aromatase inhibitors
Anastrozole

Studies comparing the aromatase inhibitor anastrozole and tamoxifen in women with breast cancer have shown that anastrozole is up to twice as effective as tamoxifen at preventing the development of new breast cancers in postmenopausal women. A current study compares anastrozole with tamoxifen in women at increased risk of breast cancer.

Letrozole and exemestane

Both letrozole and exemestane are more effective than tamoxifen at preventing new cancers in women treated for breast cancer. Prevention studies with these drugs are under way.

What should I do if I think I am at increased risk?

For a woman who believes that she is at increased risk of breast cancer the first step is to get a referral to a family history or high-risk clinic so that her individual risk can be calculated. If she is confirmed to be at significant increased risk then the following are the options:

- Regular breast checks usually with yearly mammograms and, in very high-risk women, MRI.

- Entering the new UK prevention study if she is eligible – the study is only for postmenopausal women.

- Having surgery to remove all the breast tissue. This involves some type of mastectomy on both sides. It can be combined with breast reconstruction and may or may not involve removal of the nipple. This type of surgery should be carried out by a specialist breast surgeon with or without the help of a plastic surgeon. Removal of the breasts reduces the risk of breast cancer by over 90 per cent.

- Women who are at very high risk of breast cancer because they have inherited a faulty *BRCA*-1 or

How can you best reduce your risk of developing breast cancer?

- Eat a healthy diet including regular fresh fruit and vegetables – no dietary supplements such as vitamins are necessary and no supplements have been shown to be of value

- Take regular exercise

- Drink alcohol in moderation

- Be breast aware and report any changes to your GP

- Try to keep your weight within the recommended range for your height

- Don't smoke

BRCA-2 gene are also at increased risk of ovarian cancer. Removal of the ovaries in these women not only reduces their risk of developing ovarian cancer, but also reduces their risk of developing breast cancer by half.

About half of the studies that have looked at the relationship of breast cancer and the amount of fat in a woman's diet have shown that the more fat in the diet the higher the risk of getting breast cancer. The other half, however, have not shown any clear link between a high-fat diet and breast cancer.

The current view is that it is better for your overall health to have a diet that is not high in fat so, from a general health point of view, high-fat diets are not good for you. There is some evidence that if you eat certain types of oily fish it might be beneficial.

Eating fresh fruit and vegetables is beneficial because they contain the vitamins A, C, D and E, which are known as antioxidants. They are effective at neutralising some of the substances in the environment that we think might cause cancer. Taking extra vitamins is not, however, beneficial and not recommended.

There is no convincing evidence that dairy products increase your risk of breast cancer or that avoiding dairy products will significantly decrease your risk. There is more concern about the possibility of harmful effects of soy than there is evidence of its benefits. Replacing dairy milk with soy milk is therefore not recommended unless there are medical or personal reasons for choosing soy milk.

KEY POINTS

■ Risk factors for breast cancer include female sex, increasing age and a strong family history of breast cancer

■ Taking HRT, particularly combined oestrogen and progesterone for long periods, increases the risk of breast cancer

■ There is little that one can do about most risk factors for breast cancer but it is worthwhile eating a healthy diet, taking regular exercise and avoiding HRT if possible

■ No drugs are recommended to reduce the risk of breast cancer in the general population

■ In a few women with a greatly increased risk of breast cancer due to abnormal genes, action can be taken to reduce their risk

Breast screening

Who gets screened for breast cancer?

Breast screening is a way of finding breast cancers early when they are too small for you to feel. Screening is normally carried out by using X-rays called mammograms.

Currently all women registered with a GP and aged between 50 and 69 years are offered screening by X-ray mammography every three years. Women over 69 years are not automatically invited for breast screening but these women can still have free mammograms by making an appointment every three years. Each year approximately one to one and a half million women in the UK attend for screening mammograms. Screening will be extended to include all women from 47 to 73 over the next few years.

What is a mammogram?

A mammogram is a low-dose X-ray of the breast. It is a test to look for early breast cancer.

Mammogram

A mammogram is a special kind of breast X-ray.

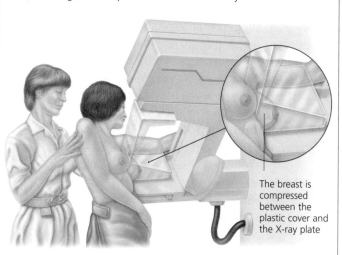

The breast is compressed between the plastic cover and the X-ray plate

How is it performed?

To have a mammogram you need to remove your clothes from only the top part of your body including your bra. Each breast is then placed on the X-ray machine in turn and gently but firmly compressed using a flat clear plastic plate and an X-ray image taken.

Benefits of screening
Finding cancer early

Most cancers diagnosed through screening are found at an early stage when there is a good chance that treatment will be successful and eradicate the cancer. In the UK, more than two-thirds of screen-detected cancers are detected at a very early stage, that is they are small and have not spread to the lymph glands.

Over 15 million women have had screening in the UK since the programme started in 1988. In that time over 85,000 cancers have been detected.

Studies suggest that screening saves at least 300 lives every year and by 2010 the number of lives saved each year may be as high as 1,000. Studies also suggest that, for every 500 women who attend for breast screening, one will have her life saved.

Less treatment is possible

Women who are found to have cancer through breast screening are more likely to have small cancers that can be treated by lumpectomy (removal of the lump) combined with postoperative radiotherapy, also called breast-conserving treatment, rather than removal of the whole breast (mastectomy).

Seventy per cent of women diagnosed with breast cancer through breast screening have breast-conserving treatment compared with 55 per cent of women whose cancer is not detected through screening.

Problems with screening
Not prevention

Screening does not prevent breast cancer. Women who are going to develop breast cancer will do so whether or not they are screened. Screening helps find cancers only if they are already there.

Pain and discomfort associated with having a mammogram

To get a good quality mammogram the breast tissue does need to be compressed (squashed). Many women find mammography uncomfortable or painful but any pain or discomfort lasts for a very short time.

Having mammograms involves more X-rays

Mammograms use only a very small dose of radiation to the breast. The amount of radiation is similar to the dose of radiation a person would receive from flying in an airplane from the UK to Australia and back. The risk from the very low dose of radiation is far outweighed by the benefits of detecting a breast cancer early.

Finding abnormalities in the breast that are not serious

Mammograms can detect a range of benign conditions as well as cancers. A woman who has an abnormal area in the breast detected on a mammogram will need to undergo more tests to show that the abnormality is not a cancer. This means that some women undergo unnecessary tests and have the worry associated with being recalled for these tests for no real benefit.

This happens with any screening programme and is known as a false-positive result. Fortunately it is not very common in breast screening.

Women recalled for extra mammograms when there is no abnormality

Some women are recalled for further mammograms because either the X-ray is blurred or the whole breast was not included on the X-ray. Nowadays, this is extremely uncommon but it is sometimes necessary to call women back to ensure that the X-ray is of sufficient quality.

Breast screening does not detect all cancers

Mammography is the best and most reliable way to detect breast cancer but it is not perfect. Breast cancer can sometimes be missed on a mammogram for a number of reasons:

- Some cancers are very difficult to see on an X-ray.

- Some cancers are there but are very small so they are not large enough to be seen on the X-ray.

- The cancer is present on the X-ray but it is missed by the person reading the mammograms.

Having mammograms every three years is the most cost-effective way of breast screening but, because the three-year gap is quite long, some women will develop breast cancer between one round of screening and the next. If you do have a cancer diagnosed during screening or between screening visits, any mammograms taken previously may be useful to your doctors.

In most cancers diagnosed between screens, when the previous mammograms are looked at there is not a significant abnormality on the previous mammogram and it is a new development, rather than the cancer having been present on the previous X-ray but having been missed by the person reading it.

Overdiagnosis

Some cancers found by breast screening are not of a problem type so that they would never have caused a problem later in life. This means that screening diagnoses cancers in some women when treatment during the patient's lifetime would never have been needed.

Unfortunately it is not possible to tell which cancers will and which will not spread and cause problems. For this reason it is better when a cancer is detected to treat it effectively even if sometimes this is over-treatment.

Organisation of screening

There are more than 90 breast screening units across the UK. All women receive their first invitation to screening some time between the ages of 50 and 53 and invitations are then sent out every three years up to and including the age of 70 years.

If you receive an invitation from your local breast-screening unit, you will be given a date, time and place to attend. This may be to one of the specialised fixed screening units across the country or to a mobile unit that looks like a large van which is usually in a convenient place such as a car park in a shopping centre.

If the appointment is inconvenient, you can telephone the breast-screening unit and they will arrange an alternative appointment. The phone number will be on the letter.

What happens when I go for screening?

A visit to a breast screening unit usually takes only about half an hour. You will be greeted by a female receptionist or a female radiographer who will check your personal details (name, age and address). The radiographer will ask you some questions about your general health and whether you have had any previous breast problems.

You will then receive an explanation of how the mammogram will be taken. Staff will be very happy to answer any questions that you have about breast screening.

Results from screening

You and your GP should get the results of the mammograms in writing within two weeks. If you do not hear anything within that time you can phone your breast-screening unit and ask them to check your results. Eleven of every twelve women who attend for screening will have a normal mammogram.

About one in twelve women who go for breast screening is asked to come back for further tests. The problem may not be cancer because there are many breast changes that can show up on a mammogram that are not serious. If you are brought back you will be invited to return to an assessment clinic and have further tests.

You will probably experience a range of emotions from anxiety to fear if you are asked to come back for further tests. It is important to remember that in seven of eight women who are recalled for assessment further tests show nothing wrong or that they have a benign condition. Only one in eight women who come back for further tests will be diagnosed as having breast cancer.

What do mammograms show?

Mammograms show normal breast tissue as white and fat as black. Anything that is abnormal also shows up as white. Cancers are classically extra blobs of white tissue with an irregular margin and are often described as stellate because they look like stars.

In fact, looking for cancers is like looking for stars at night. When the night is very cloudy, as is the situation in young women who have dense breast tissue which shows as white on the mammogram, it can be quite difficult to see stars or cancers even though they are there. When the night sky is clear, as when there is a lot of fat in the breast, which is the situation in older women, it is much easier to see the stars or cancers.

The two main reasons why screening mammograms are usually performed in women over the age of 50 years:

- The incidence of breast cancer increases with age and therefore there are more cancers in older women.

- Cancers are easier to see on the mammograms in older women. In younger women who have more active breast tissue a cancer is usually more difficult to detect.

The main types of abnormality detected through breast screening are:

- rounded masses

- irregular masses

- disturbance of architecture.

Rounded masses

These have very crisp clean edges on the mammogram and show up as an extra white blob that is separate from the surrounding breast tissue. These are most commonly benign lumps such as cysts, which are fluid filled, or fibroadenomas, which are solid, benign, localised overgrowths of breast tissue. About four per cent (4 in 100) of rounded masses turn out to be cancers.

Irregular masses

These also show up as white blobs on a mammogram. However, their edges on the mammogram are much more fuzzy and irregular. The majority of new irregular masses are cancers.

Mammography

Mammography uses low-dose X-rays to examine the human breast. The purpose of mammography is the early detection of breast cancer,

Examples of mammograms

Normal appearance of the breast of a mature, postmenopausal woman. The glandular (milk-secreting) component of the breast decreases as a woman approaches the menopause. Glandular tissue becomes replaced by fibrous connective tissue packed with fat cells. Here, fibrous tissue appears as the fine white network across the breast.

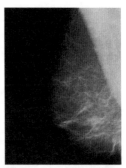

Localised mass in the breast (cancer)

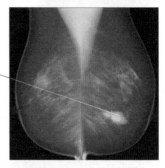

Malignant calcification indicating ductal carcinoma *in situ* (DCIS)

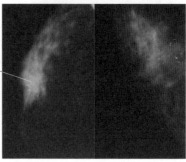

Mammography (contd)

typically through detection of unusual and characteristic masses and/or microcalcifications.

Examples of mammograms

Gross distortion in the breast with:

Malignant axillary node

Calcification (cancer)

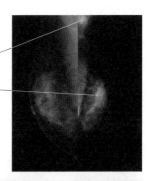

Small spiculated mass in the breast (cancer)

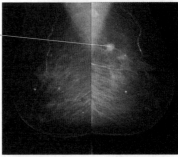

Area of distortion in the breast with microcalcification

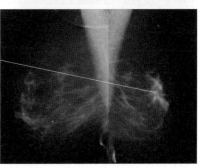

Disturbance of architecture

This is one of the most difficult abnormalities to detect. The breast tissue is pulled in around a central area so that the breast tissue around it looks distorted.

Disturbances of architecture can be benign and occur as a result of scarring or can be malignant with a cancer in the centre. Needle biopsies cannot always tell the difference between distortion caused by scarring or distortion caused by a cancer and it may be necessary to remove the area to be certain of the cause of the abnormality.

Calcifications

Small areas of calcium are common in the breast and they are often seen on mammograms. In most cases they are harmless. There are two types of calcification:

- Macrocalcifications

- Microcalcifications.

Macrocalcifications

Macrocalcifications are larger, coarse, calcium deposits in the breast that appear as white dots or dashes on a mammogram. They are the natural result of breast ageing and are found in about half of women aged over 50 and one in 10 younger women.

They may be caused by calcium deposits in cysts or by calcium building up in the milk ducts in the breast. They can also occur as a result of previous injury, surgery or radiotherapy.

These calcifications are not related to how much calcium is included in your diet. They are harmless, are not linked with cancer and do not need any treatment.

Microcalcifications

These are tiny deposits of calcium that show up as fine white specks on a mammogram. Similar to macrocalcifications, they can occur because of the ageing process in the breast, but they can also occur as a result of cells growing more quickly than normal. Usually microcalcifications are not the result of cancer.

If the microcalcifications vary in shape and size, line up within the milk ducts of the breast and have a branching pattern, these are indications that the calcifications might be the result of overgrowth or early cancerous change of the cells lining the milk ducts.

Microcalcifications seen close together or in clusters are a sign that there may be precancerous changes (see Ductal carcinoma *in situ*, page 68) in this area of the breast.

If microcalcifications are seen, you will usually be asked to have a further mammogram to look at the area in more detail (magnification mammogram). Depending on the result of this mammogram the doctor will either recommend taking no further action or advise a needle core biopsy, which involves taking a sliver of tissue from the area to remove part of the calcification so that this can be examined under the microscope (see page 53).

The problem is that a core biopsy removes only a very small amount of tissue and sometimes insufficient calcification is sampled and further tests are needed. Areas of calcification can be sampled adequately by using a slightly larger needle with suction, to suck breast tissue into the needle.

These vacuum-assisted biopsy devices remove more tissue and are easier for women because the needle has to be inserted only once into the breast. If despite all the needle tests the doctors fail to get enough calcification to be certain what is causing it, the area may need to be removed by surgery.

KEY POINTS

■ Women are offered breast screening with a breast X-ray every three years between the ages of 50 and 69

■ Breast screening aims to find cancers early when less aggressive treatment may be needed

■ Breast screening may find changes in the breast that are not serious but need extra tests to be sure that the changes are benign and not cancerous

■ Breast screening may find abnormalities in the breast that are precancerous (known as DCIS or ductal carcinoma *in situ*) which if left alone in the breast change into cancers over many months or years

Symptoms and signs of breast cancer

What are the common signs?

The symptoms of a breast cancer can include:

- a breast lump

- change of shape of the breast including dimpling of the skin

- change in the skin overlying the breast such as ulceration or discharge

- in-drawing of the nipple, called nipple inversion or nipple retraction

- changes to the surface of the nipple including eczema or scaling

- discharge from the nipple

- breast pain

- swelling and inflammation of the breast

- swelling under the arm (armpit or axilla)

- breast lumpiness.

Most women with these symptoms do not have breast cancer.

Breast lumps

A breast lump is the most common reason for women to be referred to a breast clinic. Most breast lumps are not cancer and only about one in eight lumps is malignant (cancerous).

Although most areas of lumpiness are benign (non-cancerous) and related to changes that happen in relation to the regular menstrual cycle, very occasionally lumpiness is a symptom of breast cancer. For this reason it is important that if you notice any change in the shape or feel of your breasts you get this checked by your doctor.

Cancerous lumps

Cancerous lumps tend to feel hard and tend not to be very mobile. They usually come up slowly and increase in size over time.

If the lump gets bigger, it can cause a change in the shape of the breast with puckering or dimpling of the overlying skin. If left untreated they can grow into the skin and cause ulceration or bleeding.

Benign lumps

Benign lumps tend to be smooth and mobile and move easily under the fingers. Benign lumps are also more likely to be tender whereas breast cancer tends to be painless. Common causes of benign lumps include fibroadenomas and cysts.

Fibroadenomas are benign solid lumps that are common in young women between the ages of 15 and 25. Although they are less common in older women, small fibroadenomas are often discovered in women over the age of 50 when they attend for breast screening.

Fibroadenomas tend to grow to a certain size and then stop – unlike cancers. This means that once a woman discovers a fibroadenoma it is rare for the woman to report that it continues to grow. Occasionally fibroadenomas are large and measure over five centimetres.

Provided that they are properly investigated by imaging and needle biopsy smaller fibroadenomas do not need to be removed. As large fibroadenomas cause a distortion and change in the shape of the breast, they are usually removed.

Fibroadenomas can get larger during pregnancy because they fill up with milk. A woman with a fibroadenoma is not significantly more likely to get breast cancer and cancer is not more likely to develop in a fibroadenoma than in any other part of the breast tissue.

Cysts

As the breast ages the leaves of the breast tree, the lobules, can fill up with fluid and these fluid-filled lumps are known as cysts. They are most common in women between the ages of 40 and 50 years.

Cysts usually feel very smooth and mobile but can sometimes be quite firm and hard. A woman who finds one cyst will often be shown to have more cysts when she is scanned using ultrasound.

Ultrasound can tell the difference between a cyst and a solid lump and, provided that the ultrasound shows that the lump is a simple cyst, the cyst does not need treatment unless it is causing pain or a change in the shape of the breast, when the fluid in the cyst can be drained using a needle. Cyst fluid ranges in colour from yellow to green to blue/black.

Cancers rarely develop in cysts. Ultrasound looks at the wall of the cyst so it can tell whether the cyst is innocent or if a cancer is present.

Ultrasound scan of the breast

Ultrasound passes freely through fluid and soft tissues but is reflected back when it hits a more solid (dense) surface. For example, the ultrasound wave will travel freely though healthy breast tissue, but when it hits a solid lump such as a cancer, a lot of the ultrasound waves are absorbed into the cancer and don't reflect back. A computer interprets the results to produce an image.

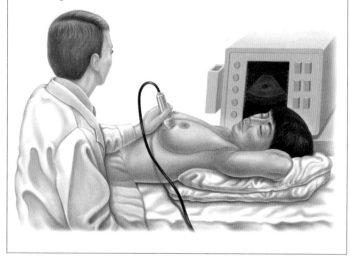

Benign localised lumpiness or nodularity

Many women's breasts get lumpy and tender just before their periods. Most localised nodularity is caused by changes that occur in relation to the normal menstrual cycle. Very rarely an area of lumpiness is the first sign of a breast cancer.

It is for this reason that, if lumpiness is confirmed at the clinic, you will have an ultrasound to check the lumpy area. Ultrasound can see through the breast tissue and tell whether a lumpy area is simply normal breast tissue that has been affected by the menstrual cycle or whether it is more serious.

Changes in the skin of the breast

This includes dimpling, puckering and swelling of the skin of the breast (known as peau d'orange or orange-peel appearance). In-drawing or puckering of the skin, also known as dimpling, is the most common skin change seen in cancer.

Occasionally the skin over a breast cancer can ulcerate and bleed. A cancer that spreads can also produce one or more nodules in the skin.

Peau d'orange develops because cancer cells block the lymph channels draining the breast and stop the normal flow of fluid out of the breast. This results in a build-up of fluid in the skin of the breast. It is sometimes associated with redness and tenderness of the breast, characteristic of a particular type of cancer called inflammatory breast cancer.

Peau d'orange and redness can also happen as a result of infection or inflammation not related to cancer.

Nipple eczema or scaling

An itchy red rash of the nipple or the areola can sometimes be a sign of an underlying cancer. This change in the nipple is known as Paget's disease and more details can be found on page 90. Most skin rashes around the nipple are not related to Paget's disease but from eczema of the skin. The biggest difference between Paget's disease and eczema is that Paget's disease always affects the nipple first whereas eczema usually first affects the area around the nipple which is known as the areola.

If the doctor decides that the condition is simple eczema, treatment is a short sharp course of steroids. Sometimes stronger steroids for a shorter duration are more successful at controlling the eczema than a more dilute steroid over a longer period of time.

Nipple inversion or retraction

The nipple can be pulled in as a consequence of disease in the breast (benign conditions or cancer) or can happen as breast ducts shorten, which they do in some women as they get older. Inversion or pulling in of the nipple does not therefore mean that a cancer is present.

If the nipple appearance does change, you should see your doctor and be referred to hospital to have a mammogram and possibly an ultrasound scan. In some women the nipple can be pulled in at certain times and at other times the nipple comes out and looks normal; this is rarely associated with cancer.

In cancer the whole nipple tends to be pulled in and it is usually pulled in one particular direction which results in the two nipples being at different heights and not pointing in the same directions. Changes associated with cancer usually involve one breast rather than both breasts.

Nipple discharge

Discharge from the nipple is very common. Even in a woman who is not pregnant, the breast produces fluid that passes up the ducts towards the nipple. This discharge does not get out onto the surface of the nipple because the ducts of the nipple are normally plugged or blocked by keratin, which is produced by the skin.

If the ducts become unplugged which can occur either because the nipple is cleaned or the nipple is squeezed, it is common to get fluid appearing on the surface of the nipple. This fluid, which varies in colour from white to yellow to green to blue/black, is normal breast secretion. There is usually a very small amount of it and it dries up very quickly.

Abnormal nipple discharge is discharge that leaks out spontaneously. It usually stains clothes and occurs on a regular basis – more than twice a week.

Sometimes the discharge can be bloody in colour or bloodstained. Even bloodstained discharge is most commonly due to a benign (non-cancerous) cause and the most common cause of a bloody discharge is a wart in one of the ducts underneath the nipple. The proper name for this is an intraduct papilloma.

Occasionally women who are not pregnant produce milk from the breast. The main cause of this is one of a series of drugs that cause an increase in the hormone that results in milk formation, called prolactin. There are lots of drugs that can do this. Occasionally a tumour in the brain develops that produces increased amounts of prolactin, which then results in milk production.

Women who are not pregnant and produce a significant amount of milky discharge or women who have discharge that is spontaneous, persistent (more than twice per week) or at all troublesome should seek medical attention.

Breast pain

This is rarely a symptom of breast cancer. In one study about five per cent of women who had cancer had pain as their main symptom and only two per cent of women who presented with breast pain were found on investigations to have a breast cancer.

Most pain in the breast does not actually originate in the breast but arises from the underlying ribs and muscles. If you have what you think is pain in the breast, it is important to check that the pain is coming from the breast and not from the area under the breast.

This is best done by turning on your side, which lets the breast roll away from the chest wall. You should then check for any tender areas in the ribs and muscles underneath the breast.

Most breast pain requires no specific treatment. Measures that improve breast pain include wearing a soft supporting bra 24 hours a day and regular gentle stretching exercise such as swimming.

Chest wall pain is common in people who sit at computers all day. It is important not to sit for longer than an hour at a time and to take a rest and have a walk. If breast pain is severe try drugs such as paracetamol or ibuprofen. If the pain does not respond to these simple measures ask your doctor for a referral to a breast clinic.

Breast swelling/inflammation

If the breast swells and becomes tender and red this is usually a sign of infection. If you are concerned that you are getting a breast infection, particularly if you are breast-feeding, it is important that you see a doctor and start antibiotics as soon as possible to stop abscess formation.

Very rarely swelling and inflammation of the breast indicate a rare form of breast cancer called inflammatory breast cancer. Despite antibiotics, in inflammatory breast cancer the swelling and redness persist. The breast can also feel painful and is tender to touch in this condition.

What are the reasons why women attend breast clinics?

Prevalence (%) of various symptoms in patients attending a breast clinic

- Breast lump 36%
- Painful lump or lumpiness 33%
- Pain alone 17.5%
- Nipple discharge 5%
- Nipple retraction 3%
- Strong family history of breast cancer 3%
- Breast distortion 1%
- Swelling or inflammation 1%
- Scaling of nipple (eczema) 0.5%

KEY POINTS

- A lump in the breast is the most common symptom of breast cancer

- Pulling in of the nipple can be a symptom of breast cancer but most cases are due to benign disease

- A change in the shape of the breast or nipple, nipple discharge, redness and a lump in the armpit are sometimes found by women who have breast cancer

- Breast pain is rarely a sign of breast cancer

- Most women with symptoms in the breast (including lumps) do not have breast cancer

Seeing your doctor

What should I do if I have breast symptoms?

Whenever you experience any symptoms relating to your breasts the first person to consult is your GP. The priority for your GP is to decide whether there is a chance that you have any serious disease within the breast and, if not, whether the problem can be sorted out without referring you to hospital.

If you have a definite lump or you have a symptom for which your doctor wishes to seek further advice, you will be referred to a hospital breast clinic. Alternatively your GP may decide that your breast should be checked again – perhaps at a different point in your menstrual cycle – and he or she will ask you to come back for a follow-up examination.

The hospital breast clinic

The doctor at the clinic will ask you to describe your symptoms in detail and also ask how long you have had them. If your problem is pain or a lump he or she will also want to know whether this varies in relation to your monthly cycle.

You will then have a breast examination. If you are seeing a male doctor he will ask for a female nurse to be present during the examination. During this examination you will be asked to strip to the waist (remove clothes from top half of body).

Physical examination

The doctor will look at your breasts first with your arms by your side, then above your head and finally with your arms pressing on your hips. By looking carefully at the outline of the breast in these various positions, the doctor may see changes that help to identify the site and cause of any problem.

Next, your breasts will be examined with you lying flat with your arms tucked underneath your head. If during the examination the doctor finds a lump, he or she may concentrate on this area, examining it with the fingertips and measuring the lump.

After checking your breasts, the doctor will usually examine the lymph glands in the armpit and those in the lower part of the neck. Should you need any further investigations, the breast specialist who sees you will order these tests and explain why these are necessary.

Mammograms (breast X-rays)

If you are over 35 years and have not had a breast X-ray within the past year the clinic doctor is likely to send you to have mammograms. For more information, see page 26.

Some breast units arrange for patients to have mammograms before they are seen by the clinic doctor so that the X-rays are reported when you see the

Breast examination by your doctor

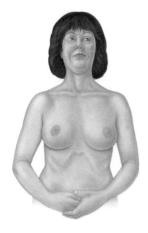

Arms to the side.

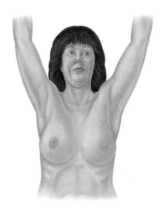

Arms over your head.

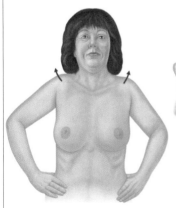

Arms on hips.

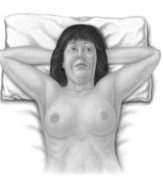

Lying down, arms folded underneath head.

Mammogram

A mammogram is a breast X-ray used to discover cancer at an early and more curable stage.

X-ray film of breast

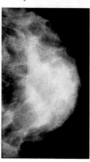

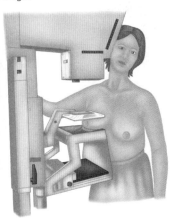

doctor. The results of the X-rays are usually ready for during the time that you are at the clinic.

Ultrasound scanning

X-rays do not pass easily through the dense breast tissue in the breasts of women under the age of 35 years and this usually makes it difficult to obtain images of sufficiently good quality in younger women. In these women and in older women with a lump an extra test called an ultrasound scan may be performed.

Ultrasound is familiar to many women because it is used to look at babies during pregnancy. It is used in the breast to tell whether any lump is filled with fluid (cystic) or whether it is solid.

A special gel is spread on to the breast and a small device that emits high-frequency sound waves is passed over the area. The echoes are converted into a picture of the breast tissue by a computer. This scan is painless and takes just a few minutes.

Ultrasound is not useful as a screening test but is useful to investigate an abnormality on the X-ray or to assess a localised area of lumpiness. If the lump is solid on ultrasound it is usually possible to tell whether it is a benign (non-cancerous) lump, or likely to be more serious.

Ultrasound is also a very good way of looking at the lymph glands under the arm. It is now routine practice for women suspected of having breast cancer to have an ultrasound of the lymph glands under the arm. If any abnormal lymph glands are seen, these can be sampled with a small needle using the ultrasound to guide the needle into the lymph node.

Needle tests

There are two types of needle test commonly used to diagnose breast lumps.

Core biopsy

The most commonly used takes a small sliver or portion of tissue and is known as a core biopsy. Before this test is carried out the skin and the area surrounding the lump or abnormality are numbed with local anaesthetic. Provided that sufficient local anaesthetic is injected into the breast and left for several minutes to work, it is not a painful test.

When the anaesthetic wears off, however, the breast can be tender and patients are usually advised to take painkillers, similar to those used for headaches such as paracetamol or ibuprofen.

Core biopsy

A special hollow needle is inserted into the suspicious area of the patient's breast to obtain a tissue sample for analysis. This will assist the diagnosis of a lump in the breast as benign or malignant (cancerous), and then allow further treatment to be planned.

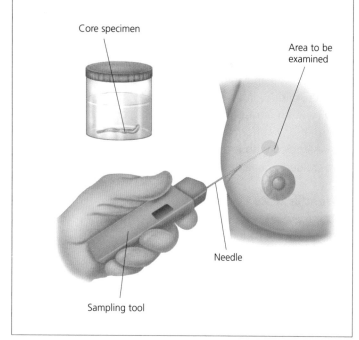

Core specimen

Area to be examined

Needle

Sampling tool

Fine-needle aspiration

The other needle test uses a small fine needle of the same size as that used to take blood; this is called fine-needle aspiration. This test removes a sample of cells. It can be performed either with or without a local anaesthetic. In some clinics results from this needle test are available within an hour.

Fine-needle aspiration

The principles are the same as for core biopsy but a finer needle is used – so the sample harvested is not as great.

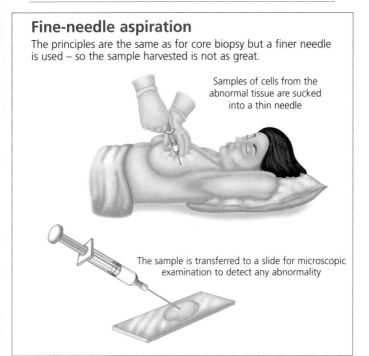

Samples of cells from the abnormal tissue are sucked into a thin needle

The sample is transferred to a slide for microscopic examination to detect any abnormality

After core biopsy or fine-needle aspiration the area may become bruised and swollen. Both a core biopsy and a fine-needle test can be carried out in the clinic or the X-ray or radiology department. In small lumps or small areas of abnormality detected on scans or X-rays, a needle can be guided into the problem area using X-ray or ultrasound guidance to make sure that the correct area is sampled. Your doctor will discuss with you what type of needle biopsy you need and exactly how the test will be carried out.

Usually the doctor at the breast clinic is able to tell you at your first clinic visit whether the lump is benign or could be more serious.

Vacuum-assisted biopsy

The predominant reason why an accurate diagnosis is not obtained by core biopsy is a failure to sample the right area or failure to obtain sufficient tissue. These problems can be largely overcome by using a larger needle with the addition of suction or a vacuum to take more tissue.

Vacuum-assisted biopsies are better at sampling calcification than core biopsy and allow biopsy of more awkward areas in the breast.

Local anaesthetic solution is injected into the skin and the breast and left in place for a few minutes to work. A small cut is then made in the skin and the needle for the biopsy is introduced into the breast. Most vacuum-assisted biopsy devices need to be inserted into the breast once only which is a distinct advantage over core needles, which need to be removed from the breast after each core to remove the sample from the needle.

As vacuum-assisted biopsies can remove most of an area of calcification, the doctor performing the biopsy may leave a metal marker in the breast at the site where the biopsy has been performed. This means that, if the area needs to be removed at operation, it is possible to find the area accurately using the metal marker as a guide.

Needle localisation biopsy

To remove an area of concern within the breast, which cannot be felt by the surgeon as a lump, it is necessary to mark this area using a thin wire with a hook at one end. Before surgery you will go down to the X-ray department and after injection of local anaesthetic a wire is placed into the breast using either the mammogram machine or ultrasound to guide it to the area that is to be removed.

After placement of a wire, X-rays are taken to check the position of the wire in relation to the area that is to be removed. Sometimes two wires are inserted either because the first wire was not inserted in a satisfactory position or because there are two areas of abnormality that need to be marked, or two wires are placed, one at each end of the abnormality, to help the surgeon remove the whole of the correct area.

When the wire(s) are in a satisfactory position you return to the ward where you are usually given something to make you feel sleepy (a pre-med). Later in the day you are taken to the operating theatre and have the operation under general anaesthetic.

A small cut is made in the skin of the breast and the surgeon finds the wire and follows it to the area of abnormality. The area of breast tissue around the wire is then removed by the surgeon. While you are still under the anaesthetic an X-ray is taken of the tissue sampled to check that the correct area has been removed.

There are other techniques that can be used to mark an abnormal area, one of which is to inject a radioactive substance into the breast around the abnormal area. The surgeon then uses a hand-held probe in the operating theatre, which detects radioactivity and allows the abnormal area to be identified and removed.

Open biopsy/excision biopsy

It used to be common to remove a lump by surgery to find out what it was (an open or excision biopsy).

Nowadays it is rarely necessary to remove a lump or an abnormal area on mammogram or on screening to find out its exact cause. It is usually possible with needle tests to diagnose what the lesion is. Most women who are informed that a lump or abnormalities detected in their breasts are benign do not request removal, but some women do wish to have their lump removed.

If either the doctor has advised you to have a lump removed or you have decided to have it removed, this is usually performed under a general anaesthetic, although it can be performed using a local anaesthesia.

Follow-up visits

If you do not receive the results of all your tests on the same day as they are performed you will be given a follow-up appointment to come back to get the results. Sometimes the results of the tests do not provide a definite answer, in which case you may have to have further investigations.

If a core biopsy or fine-needle aspirate has not shown a definite cause for the lump it is possible at your second visit that the doctor will suggest that the lump should be removed (an excision biopsy or needle localisation biopsy – see above).

What the tests mean

Needle tests are very accurate and are rarely ever wrong if they show cancer. Occasionally the mammogram or ultrasound scan is reported as showing a cancer but, when tested with a needle or removed, it turns out to be non-cancerous.

This might happen in 1 of 20 cases. This is why the doctor will often tell you that the lump might be cancer but it is impossible to be absolutely sure until the lump has been tested with a needle or until the lump has been removed and analysed. The combination of:

- performing a careful examination

- taking X-rays and/or scans

- performing a needle test of the lump

is very accurate. It is known as triple assessment or the triple test.

If you have all these three tests it is very rare, if a cancer is present, for it to be missed. If all the tests show that the lump is not serious, it is not therefore necessary to have the lump removed and you can be safely reassured and discharged.

Other tests that may be performed
Bone scan

Sometimes a bone scan is performed in a patient with a breast cancer to check that there is no abnormality in the bones.

For this scan a very small amount of mildly radioactive liquid is injected into a vein, usually in your arm. After the injection you will have to wait for two or three hours before the radioactivity gets to the bone, so you may want to take a book or magazine with you. Taking a friend for company is also worthwhile. The radioactive material injected is completely safe and quickly loses activity. It disappears from the body within a few hours.

A scan is then taken. Abnormal bone takes up more of the radioactive substance than normal bone and abnormalities show up on the scan as a bright area or hot spot.

Bone scan

This shows up any abnormal areas of bone in any part of the body. For this test a small amount of a radioactive substance is injected into a vein, usually in the arm, a few hours before the scan. If there is anything wrong it will be shown up by an increased uptake of the radioactive substance in the affected area.

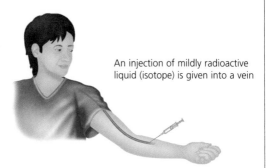

An injection of mildly radioactive liquid (isotope) is given into a vein

You will be asked to lie under a special camera that can detect the isotope in your body

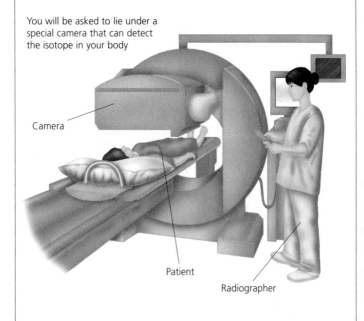

Camera

Patient

Radiographer

Areas of previous injury or arthritis can also show up on the scan as hot spots. To sort out whether a hot spot is related to previous injury you may be asked to have further X-rays of these areas. If there is a hot spot and there is evidence of damage to the bone, this might indicate that this is related to cancer that has spread to the bones.

Magnetic resonance imaging

This test does not use X-rays but magnetism to build up a picture of your body. It can be used to look at the breasts or other areas of the body, particularly bones.

This is a difficult test if you suffer from claustrophobia. During the scan you will be asked to lie very still on a couch inside a long chamber for up to 40 minutes. If you cannot lie in enclosed spaces you should mention this to your doctor or the radiographer when you attend for the scan.

Magnetic resonance imaging (MRI) is also very noisy but you will be given earplugs or headphones to reduce the noise. Some MRI departments invite you to bring your own music with you to listen to while you are having your MRI done. It is also usually possible for you to take somebody with you to keep you company.

As the scan chamber is a very powerful magnet, before entering the room you need to remove all metal belongings. People who have pacemakers or certain surgical pins or clips should not have an MR scan, so you need to tell your doctor if you have any.

Breast MRI

MR scans of the breast are very accurate but they take a long time to perform so they are used only in certain groups of women. They are very accurate at looking at

Magnetic resonance imaging (MRI)

Magnetic resonance imaging uses powerful magnets to align the atoms in the part of the body being studied. Radiowave pulses break the alignment causing signals to be emitted from the atoms. These signals can be measured and a detailed image built up of the tissues and organs.

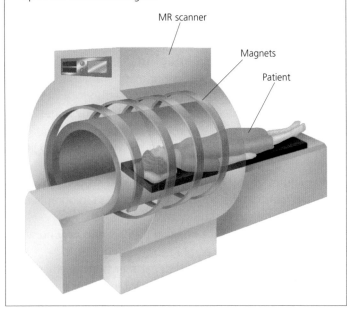

MR scanner

Magnets

Patient

young women's breasts and are particularly useful for looking at the breasts of young women who have a very strong family history of breast cancer.

Breast MRI is also valuable in women who have a lump under their arm which is shown to contain cancer cells that have spread to a lymph node, but where there is no obvious abnormality in the breast on X-rays or an ultrasound scan. MRI can sometimes find a cancer in the breast that has been missed by other tests.

In women who have had surgery and/or radiotherapy to the breast MR scans are particularly useful. Surgery and radiotherapy can cause scarring and it can be difficult on X-ray to be certain whether an abnormality in the breast of a woman who has had previous surgery and radiotherapy is the result of scarring or there is a more serious abnormality present.

MRI is also the best way of getting a picture of woman's breasts that have breast implants in place. If there is concern that an implant is leaking or ruptured, MRI is the best way of telling whether the implant is intact or leaking.

Whole body MRI

Sorting out whether an abnormality on a bone scan is related to a previous injury or arthritis, or spread from a cancer, is not always easy and MR scans are a very accurate way of looking at bone. They are sometimes needed in patients with hot spots on bone scans to determine whether there is a serious cause for the bone scan abnormality.

MR scans of the liver, brain and spinal cord are useful in women with breast cancer who develop symptoms to suggest that there may be an abnormality in these areas.

Ultrasound scan of the liver

In women with larger cancers, where there are signs that the liver is not functioning normally, or where tests have shown spread to the bone or lungs, a liver ultrasound scan or CT scan of the liver can help to assess whether cancer has spread to the liver. If you are asked to have an ultrasound scan to check your liver this is a painless test and takes only a few minutes.

It will probably be done in the hospital scanning department. You will be asked to lie on a couch, a gel will be spread on to your tummy and a small device that sends out sound waves will be passed over the area. The echo of the sound waves is converted into a picture by a computer.

CT scan of the liver

If ultrasound does not get a very good picture of the liver, the doctor may suggest that you have a CT scan. CT stands for computed tomography. It uses X-rays to build up a picture of what the body looks like at one particular level in the body. By taking these pictures at multiple levels it is possible to get a very accurate picture of the liver and see if there are any abnormalities in it. In some units CT scans of the liver are preferred to ultrasound scans.

Computed tomography is also used for looking at other areas of the body, including the lungs, bone and brain. It can help to show whether any abnormality on an X-ray or ultrasound scan is due to spread from the breast cancer.

Positron emission tomography

Commonly known as PET, this technique relies on the fact that cancers grow faster than normal cells. By using labelled glucose, which is a fuel for cells, those cells that are growing faster take up more glucose and therefore show up as abnormal on these scans.

This allows breast cancers that have spread to be seen on the PET scan. The main problem with PET is that it is very expensive and available only in certain centres. It can be combined with CT and is then known as CTPET.

Computed tomography (CT)

Computed tomography fires X-rays through the body at different angles. The X-rays are picked up by receivers and the information analysed by a computer to create a picture of the body.

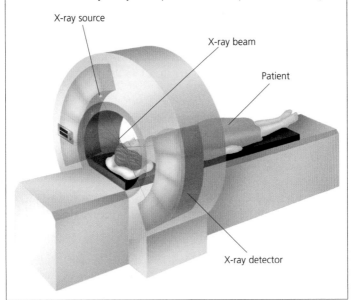

X-ray source

X-ray beam

Patient

X-ray detector

It is also not clear whether PET scans provide any additional benefit for patients with breast problems compared with the other investigations already widely available in most hospitals.

KEY POINTS

- If your GP thinks that you have significant breast symptoms he or she will refer you to a hospital breast clinic

- At the hospital breast clinic various tests will be carried out to determine the cause of the symptoms

- These tests commonly include physical examination of the breast area, a mammogram, scans and needle (biopsy) tests

- It is usually possible to establish a definite diagnosis of a lump or X-ray abnormality by a needle test performed after injecting local anaesthetic

- Other tests can check for possible areas to which a cancer may spread including the bone (bone scan) and liver (liver ultrasound)

Stages and types of breast cancer

Are there different types of breast cancer?
Many women do not realise that breast cancer is not just one disease that is treated in a standard way with the same predictable outlook for each person who gets it. There are many different types of breast cancer and there are many aspects of this disease that play a part in determining the best treatment and whether the outlook is likely to be better or worse than for another patient with the disease.

Factors that need to be considered include:

- The size of the tumour

- What the tumour looks like under the microscope

- Whether there has been spread to the lymph nodes

- Whether the cancer is hormone sensitive

- Whether the cancer has certain growth factors on its surface or whether the cancer is HER2 positive.

Breast cancer can be classified into two main types:

- Non-invasive

- Invasive.

Non-invasive cancers

Breast cancers develop from the cells that line the breast lobules (leaves of the breast tree) and draining ducts (or branches). Cancer cells that are confined to the lobules and ducts are called *in situ* or non-invasive.

These are sometimes referred to as pre-cancer and can be split into two types based on their appearance under the microscope. The two types are:

1 Ductal carcinoma *in situ* (DCIS)

2 Lobular carcinoma *in situ* (LCIS).

Another term for LCIS is lobular neoplasia.

It was thought originally that lobular carcinoma *in situ* arose in the lobules (leaves of the breast tree) and ductal carcinoma *in situ* arose in the ducts (branches of breast tree). We now know that this is not true, in that all cancers arise in the lobule alone or in the final branch of the ducts and the lobule, the so-called terminal duct lobular unit.

Ductal carcinoma *in situ* (DCIS)

This condition is often referred to by its initials, DCIS, rather than the full name ductal carcinoma *in situ*. The cells lining the milk ducts that carry the milk to the nipple can overgrow to such an extent that they look cancerous, but they remain confined to the milk duct channels.

DCIS is sometimes called pre-invasive, non-invasive or intraductal cancer. It used to be quite rare but has

Non-invasive or precancerous cells

Ductal carcinoma *in situ* (DCIS) is an early form of breast cancer, sometimes described as an intraductal or non-invasive cancer. This means that the cancer cells are inside the milk ducts (terminal duct lobular unit) or *in situ* and have not developed the ability to spread through the breast or outside it. There are a number of different types of DCIS.

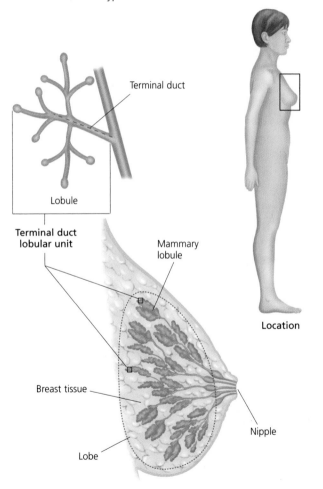

Terminal duct

Lobule

Terminal duct lobular unit

Mammary lobule

Breast tissue

Lobe

Nipple

Location

become much more common since the introduction of breast screening. Although DCIS can sometimes present as a lump, most women with DCIS have no signs or symptoms and they only know that they have it because it has been found on a mammogram.

DCIS usually shows on the mammogram as a localised area of microcalcification and the flecks of calcium are very small. Occasionally women with DCIS find a breast lump or have nipple discharge.

If DCIS is left untreated it is likely that, as time passes, cancer cells will spread and invade from the ducts into the surrounding tissue to form a true invasive cancer. Although DCIS should be treated to stop it developing into invasive cancer, provided that it is removed completely, it cannot cause any harm.

Not every woman who has DCIS will go on to develop invasive cancer. There are different types of DCIS and they can be separated into different groups based on the cell pattern and appearance under the microscope.

The most common classification is into three groups based on the resemblance of the cells in the DCIS to the normal cells lining the milk ducts. These three groups are:

1 low grade

2 intermediate grade

3 high grade.

Low-grade DCIS

These cells resemble normal cells in many ways, although they are clearly abnormal. They have the slowest rate of growth.

Intermediate-grade DCIS

These cells have some features of normal cells. They have a growth rate between that of low-grade and high-grade DCIS.

High-grade DCIS

The DCIS cells in this group are larger and do not resemble the normal cells lining the milk ducts. They have the highest growth rate and have a tendency to be larger than other types of DCIS. They also sometimes outgrow their blood supply and so some areas within the DCIS die – this is called necrosis.

After removal of an area of low-grade DCIS there appears to be a low rate of the DCIS coming back and a low rate of development of cancer in the same area of the breast. In comparison, high-grade DCIS is more likely to recur after removal and is more likely to develop into an invasive cancer than low-grade DCIS if left untreated.

If a cancer develops in an area of low-grade DCIS it is likely to be a low-grade (less aggressive) cancer. One that develops after the treatment of a high-grade DCIS tends to be a high-grade (worse than low-grade) invasive cancer.

How is DCIS treated?

Surgery is the main treatment for DCIS. Provided that all the DCIS is removed from the breast, this should be a cure.

Breast-conserving surgery

If the DCIS is localised to a small portion of the breast,

breast-conserving surgery (complete removal of the DCIS with some surrounding normal tissue) is usually possible.

With breast-conserving surgery alone there is a risk that further DCIS or an invasive cancer will develop in future and this most commonly occurs in breast tissue immediately at the edge of where the surgery has been performed.

Radiotherapy

For this reason most women with DCIS who have breast-conserving surgery are advised to have radiotherapy after their surgery because this markedly reduces the risks of further disease developing in the breast. There are some women, however, with small low- and intermediate-grade cancers who are satisfactorily treated by breast-conserving surgery to remove the DCIS alone.

Mastectomy

Although breast-conserving surgery is possible for small and medium-sized areas of DCIS, if there is more extensive disease in the breast over an area of more than four centimetres, or more than one area of the breast is affected by DCIS, then a mastectomy is usually advised.

Patients with DCIS who have a mastectomy are ideal candidates for breast reconstruction. Patients can have skin-sparing mastectomy where most of the skin is left intact and the scars from surgery are kept to a minimum.

If a mastectomy is performed, the surgeon will often remove some of the lymph glands in the armpit to check that the nodes are clear. To identify the lymph glands that are most likely to be affected a procedure called sentinel node biopsy (see page 116) is performed.

The reason is that, when a large area of DCIS is removed, and examined under the microscope, there will occasionally be small areas where the cancer has become invasive. Checking the lymph glands and knowing that these are clear means that the cancer is very unlikely to have spread beyond the breast.

This armpit surgery does not significantly increase the likelihood of developing problems after the operation, but it does avoid having to go back for a second operation in those women where invasion is identified after examination of the tissue removed by the surgeon.

There is conflicting evidence whether tamoxifen is beneficial for women with DCIS. Currently studies are under way to see whether the new aromatase inhibitors (see page 142) can help in this condition. It does appear likely that tamoxifen reduces the chances of more DCIS or invasive cancer developing in women who have hormone receptor-positive DCIS.

Lobular carcinoma *in situ* (LCIS) or lobular neoplasia

Lobular neoplasia, also known as lobular intraepithelial neoplasia (LIN), is the new term that is used to include two conditions that were considered separately:

1 atypical lobular hyperplasia

2 lobular carcinoma *in situ*.

This condition is diagnosed by the pathologist after a breast biopsy. Normally only one layer of cells lines the breast lobule. When there are two or more layers of cells this is called hyperplasia. As the number of layers of cells increase the breast lobule expands and increases in size. When the whole lobule and draining ducts are expanded by abnormal round or regular cells the pathologist considers this to be lobular neoplasia. It is much less common than DCIS.

This is not a cancer but its presence in the breast means that there is an increased risk of developing breast cancer later in life. Even with this increased risk most women who have lobular neoplasia do not develop breast cancer.

It is not necessary to remove all the lobular neoplasia because what lobular neoplasia tells us is that the person is at increased risk of getting breast cancer, but any cancer that does develop can occur anywhere in either breast. For this reason careful follow-up is recommended with regular mammograms for 10 to 15 years.

Patients with lobular neoplasia are also suitable for some of the clinical trials looking at drugs to try to prevent breast cancer. In an American study, patients who had lobular neoplasia and took tamoxifen for five years halved their risk of developing breast cancer over this period.

How is lobular neoplasia diagnosed?
Lobular neoplasia is usually discovered as a chance finding in a woman who has had a breast biopsy of a lump or an abnormality detected by screening. Sometimes lobular neoplasia can cause calcification but it is most often found by chance when a breast biopsy is looked at under the microscope.

How is lobular neoplasia treated?
Most women with lobular neoplasia do not require any treatment. Only if you have lobular neoplasia and a

very strong family history of breast cancer will your doctor suggest further surgery.

As women with lobular neoplasia are at increased risk of breast cancer, regular screening is recommended, usually once a year for 10 to 15 years after the diagnosis.

Invasive cancers

A cancer is classified as invasive if the cells have moved beyond the ducts and lobules into the surrounding tissue. Non-invasive cancer can develop into invasive cancer if left untreated.

Invasive cancers have the ability to spread locally in the breast and they may enter lymph channels in the breast and spread to lymph glands, usually under the arm; this is the most common place that breast cancer spreads to.

Sometimes invasive cancers cells get into the bloodstream, either from the lymph nodes or by direct growth into blood vessels in the breast. Once in the bloodstream they can spread to any part of the body, the bones, lung, liver and brain being most commonly affected.

There are different ways of classifying invasive cancers; the one that is in most common use splits cancers into:

1 Special type tumours: the special type of invasive breast cancers include:

   ● tubular

   ● cribriform

   ● mucinous or mucoid

How cancer spreads

Cancerous tumours can spread to distant sites in the body by a process called metastasis. In metastasis the cancerous cell separates from a malignant tumour and travels to a new location in the blood or lymph.

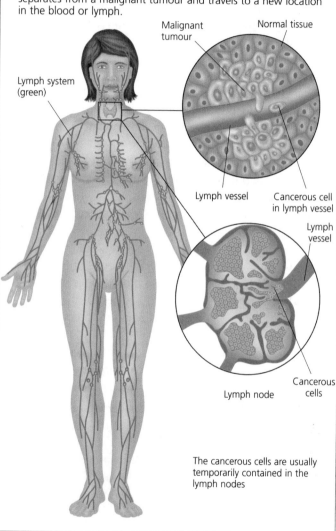

Malignant tumour

Normal tissue

Lymph system (green)

Lymph vessel

Cancerous cell in lymph vessel

Lymph vessel

Lymph node

Cancerous cells

The cancerous cells are usually temporarily contained in the lymph nodes

- papillary

- medullary

- lobular

2 Tumours of no special type (NST), also called invasive ductal cancers.

Special types of tumours
Invasive tubular cancer
This is an uncommon type of cancer. About two to three per cent of breast cancers are of this type. It is much more commonly found in women whose cancer is diagnosed through screening.

The cancer under the microscope consists of tubes of cells, which is why it gets its name. Tubular cancer has a very good outlook and few people ever die as a result of this type of cancer. As it has a very good outlook, it usually requires less treatment and women with this type of cancer almost never need chemotherapy.

Invasive cribriform cancer
This is even rarer than tubular cancer. The pattern under the microscope is rather like Swiss cheese with groups of cells and lots of holes in the centre. These cancers are very closely related to invasive tubular cancers and have the same excellent outlook.

Invasive mucinous or mucoid cancer
In this type of tumour the cancer cells produce a thick jelly-like material called mucin. These cancers are usually well rounded on X-ray and are slightly more common in older women.

They have a very good outlook. Sometimes, however, if left untreated they can become quite large. They are also known as colloid cancers.

Papillary cancers
These cancers have finger-like projections, which are lined by the cancer cells. As with medullary and mucinous cancers, they can sometimes appear as very well-defined lumps with smooth edges. Sometimes it can be difficult to tell whether these cancers are invasive or not. Women with this type of cancer tend to do better than women with cancers of no special type.

Invasive medullary cancer
This type of cancer is uncommon in women who have no family history of breast cancer but is more common in women who carry a *BRCA*-1 gene mutation. They tend to be soft and rounded lumps in the breast.

They are not always easy to pick up on X-ray and have some of the appearances of a benign lump on mammogram. Women with medullary cancers tend to have a slightly better outlook than women who have cancers of no special type.

Invasive lobular cancer
Between five and ten per cent of all cancers are classified by the pathologist as of invasive lobular type. They are called lobular because it was thought that this type of cancer arose in the lobules, whereas ordinary cancers of no special type (also called invasive ductal cancers) were thought to arise in the ducts.

It is now known that this is incorrect and all cancers arise from within the terminal duct lobular unit. Invasive lobular cancers are, however, still classified separately and the old name persists because not only do they look very different under the microscope, but they also behave differently to cancers or cancers of no special type.

In invasive lobular cancer the cancer cells push through normal tissue with the cells spreading in lines that are interspaced between the normal breast tissue. Rather than forming a lump, this type of spread often forms just a thickening.

Invasive lobular carcinoma (ILC) is a type of cancer that surgeons find most difficult to diagnose. It is much more difficult to feel and the edges of the cancer are difficult to define. They do not always show up on mammograms and needle tests can sample the normal tissue and miss the cancerous cells in between. ILC also tends to cast less of a shadow on ultrasound than cancers of no special type.

For all these reasons invasive lobular cancers are often larger at diagnosis than cancers of no special type. As a result of this, invasive lobular cancers have often also spread to lymph glands by the time that a diagnosis is made.

It is not always possible to tell how large an invasive lobular cancer is by examining the lump and this can be a problem for the surgeon because he or she may think that the cancer is small and localised, but when the surgeon tries to remove the lump they find that the cancer is more extensive.

In almost half of patients with invasive lobular cancer who have a lumpectomy, further surgery is needed to get all the cancer out. MRI is sometimes helpful at estimating the extent of disease.

Patients with invasive lobular cancer are thought to have a slightly higher risk than average of developing a cancer in the opposite breast compared with patients whose cancers are of no special type.

Cancers of no special type (also known as invasive ductal cancers)

Most cancers, approximately 85 per cent, are classified as invasive cancers of no special type, and they are commonly called invasive ductal cancers because they were thought to arise in the ducts, in contrast to invasive lobular cancer which was thought to arise in the lobule.

It is unfortunate that, when pathologists decided to give names, they used terms that we now know are not an accurate reflection of the origin of the different cancer types.

There is a whole range of cancers of no special type and they can be split into groups based on their grade (that is, how abnormal the cells look under the microscope) and whether they have receptors for hormones and certain growth factors on their surface.

Different types of invasive cancers of no special type
Rather than being one disease, invasive breast cancers of no special type are a range of different diseases. It is probably easier to explain if you compare breast cancers with dogs.

At one end of the spectrum there are small low-grade tumours that have an excellent outlook and will rarely if ever kill; these cancer cells look similar to normal breast cells which is why they are classified as low grade or grade 1, and these cancers behave much like a small well-trained family pet.

At the other end of the spectrum there are large cancers that have spread and cause problems elsewhere in the body, which look very different from normal cells and are considered high grade or grade 3 under the microscope and often grow quickly; these cancers behave more like an untrained rottweiler.

These large grade 3 cancers are still treatable and modern-day treatments can be very effective. Aggressive cancers often respond very well to treatments such as chemotherapy. The aim is to find out about your individual tumour and then tailor the treatment to suit you and your cancer.

Hormone and growth factor receptors

The hormones oestrogen and progesterone play important roles in breast cancer. Oestrogen receptors, called ERs after the American spelling of estrogen, are present in approximately 75 per cent of breast cancers. ER is expressed in much greater amounts in cancer cells than in normal breast cancer tissue. ER is thus an important target for treatment and depriving cancer cells of oestrogen causes the cancer cells to stop growing, and the cancer will eventually shrink. The majority of cancers that express ER also have receptors for progesterone and these are called PgRs. The presence of ER and PgR indicates that the cancer is likely to benefit from removing oestrogen compared with a cancer that has no ER or PgR (ER and PgR negative), where there is no benefit from hormone treatment.

Growth factors in cancer cells control the rate of growth of the cancer. The most important group of growth factors are the human epidermal growth factor receptors, also known as the HER group. There are four HER receptors, the most important of which is HER2. Blocking HER2 with a new type of drug called trastuzumab (see page 161), also known as Herceptin, reduces growth and leads to cancers shrinking and in some patients results in eradication of the cancer. About 15 to 20 per cent of all cancers have a lot of HER2 receptors and thus rely on HER2, and are candidates for treatment with trastuzumab. Treatments that block HER1 have been developed. A new oral drug, lapatanib (see page 162), blocks HER1 and HER2 together and pertuzumab (see page 162) blocks HER1, HER2 and HER3.

Currently all breast cancers are checked for ER and HER2. Some breast units routinely check for PgR but some check for PgR only in ER-negative cancers to make sure that they are not likely to benefit from hormone treatment. The amount of ER is reported as well as a simple ER positive (+ve) or ER negative (–ve). A commonly used scale classified both ER and PgR between 0 and 8. Zero is negative. There is no score of 1, the score 2 indicating a very low level of receptors. Most cancers have high levels of ER or PgR and have scores of 6, 7 or 8. Cancers with scores of 6, 7 or 8 are known as ER rich.

HER2 is reported as positive or negative but two tests are needed in borderline cases and it can sometimes take 10 to 14 days to get a HER2 result.

Cancers are classified as hormone sensitive, which means that they are ER+, PgR+; there are few if any ER–, PgR+ cancers. About 20 per cent of cancers are hormone resistant, that is they are ER–, PgR– cancers. Cancers are considered triple negative (ER–, PgR–, HER2–) if all three markers are negative on testing. Triple-negative cancers, which are often seen in women carrying an abnormal *BRCA*-1 gene (see page 210), tend to have a worse outcome, although about half do respond very well to chemotherapy.

HER2-positive cancers used to have a worse outlook than HER2-negative cancers before the widespread use of trastuzumab. This drug dramatically improves outcome in HER2-positive disease so that there is now little difference in prognosis between patients with HER2+ and those with HER2– cancers.

Lymphatic system and lymph node spread

The lymph system is a network of lymph channels and glands involved in fighting off infection. If a germ gets into the body it passes through the lymph channels to the lymph glands where the cells that are involved in killing the germs are stored.

The white blood cells in the lymph glands either kill the germs themselves or produce substances called antibodies, which are released into the bloodstream to kill the germs.

The main flow of lymph from the breast is to the lymph glands under the arm. The area under the arm is called the axilla and the lymph glands under the arm are called the axillary lymph glands or axillary lymph nodes.

It is important to know whether a cancer is localised to the breast or whether it has spread to the lymph glands or other parts of the body. Doctors describe cancers by their extent of spread and classify breast cancer into stages. Another more simple classification is to separate breast cancer into three groups:

- early breast cancer

- locally advanced breast cancer

- metastatic breast cancer.

Lymphatic drainage within the breast

Blood and lymph vessels form a network throughout each breast. Breast tissue is drained by lymphatic vessels that lead to axillary nodes and internal mammary nodes (which lie along each side of the breast bone). This is important in terms of breast cancer, as cancer cells can break away from the main tumour and may spread to other parts of the body through the lymphatic system.

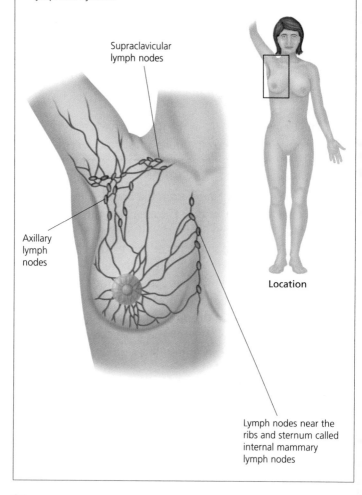

Supraclavicular lymph nodes

Axillary lymph nodes

Location

Lymph nodes near the ribs and sternum called internal mammary lymph nodes

Early breast cancer

This is cancer that is confined to the breast and/or the lymph nodes of the armpit on the same side of the body.

Locally advanced cancer

This is cancer that has not apparently spread beyond the breast and armpit but has a series of signs to suggest that it is not suited to treatment initially by surgery.

In locally advanced breast cancer either the skin of the breast is abnormal and swollen or red, or the cancer is growing directly into the skin or the muscles and ribs of the chest wall.

If these cancers are treated by surgery alone, this treatment will be successful only in less than half of patients at controlling the cancer and stopping spread to the rest of the body. In the other half the cancer comes back despite the surgery, often in areas next to where the surgery was performed.

These cancers are usually best treated by drug therapy to shrink the cancer, followed by surgery and/or radiotherapy.

Metastatic breast cancer

This is cancer that has spread beyond the breast and armpit or to other parts of the body, such as the bones, liver, lungs and even the brain. These cancers are best treated by drugs that reach cancer cells wherever they are in the body sometimes combined with local radiotherapy.

Staging

Breast cancer can be grouped into stages – commonly called staging – and there are five main stages ranging from stage 0 to stage 4. This groups cancers together that have a similar risk and very often similar treatment.

Stage 0: very early disease

This stage indicates that there is only non-invasive cancer in the breast such as DCIS or Paget's disease (see page 90) together with underlying DCIS. Stage 0 therefore includes only carcinoma *in situ*.

There are two types of stage 0 disease or carcinoma *in situ*:

1 Ductal carcinoma *in situ* known as DCIS, sometimes called intraductal carcinoma, non-invasive cancer or pre-cancer

2 Lobular cancer *in situ* (LCIS), sometimes also called lobular neoplasia.

The abnormal cells in stage 0 disease have not spread outside the duct or the lobule to invade the surrounding breast tissue.

Stage 1: early disease

To classify as stage 1:

- the cancer has to measure less than two centimetres across (approximately three-quarters of an inch)

- the cancer is localised to the breast; this means that it has not spread to the lymph glands or anywhere else in the body.

Stage 2: early disease

To classify as stage 2:

- the tumour must measure less than two centimetres across and have spread to the axillary lymph glands or

- the tumour must measure between two and five centimetres and the lymph glands may or may not be involved or

- the tumour must measure larger than five centimetres (two inches) but have no evidence of spread to the lymph glands under the arm.

Stage 3: locally advanced breast cancer

To qualify as stage 3 there must be no evidence of spread beyond:

- the skin overlying the breast

- the lymph node areas

- the chest wall.

This stage is split into three groups: stages 3a, 3b and 3c.

Stage 3a

- The tumour in the breast must be smaller than five centimetres, and the cancer has spread to the lymph glands under the arm and grown beyond the edges of the lymph gland into the surrounding tissues, such as the underlying muscles or the skin, so that the lymph glands are stuck to these tissues or

- The tumour must measure over five centimetres and the lymph glands under the arm are affected, or stuck to surrounding tissues.

Stage 3b

- The tumour must have grown directly into the skin overlying the breast, which can result in an ulcer or bleeding or

- The tumour must have grown from the breast to involve the underlying muscles and ribs of the chest wall or

- The tumour must have spread to the lymph glands under the breast bone – known as the internal mammary nodes – or

- An inflammatory breast cancer is present. This is a rare of type cancer. The next section in this chapter describes this condition (see page 89). Inflammatory cancer is diagnosed when the breast is red, swollen and inflamed. The cancer cells from these inflammatory cancers block lymph channels that drain fluid from the breast; this causes a reaction in the tissues which results in the local redness and inflammation.

Stage 3c

- The lymph glands under the breast bone and under the arm are affected by spread from the cancer or

- The lymph glands above the collar bone, known as the supraclavicular nodes, are involved with cancer.

Stage 4: metastatic disease

Stage 4 is when the cancer has metastasised (spread) beyond the breast and axillary nodes to other parts of the body. Patients sometimes but not commonly have stage 4 disease when they first present to hospital.

If the cancer returns it is usually in some other part of the body and many years after apparently effective treatment for breast cancer.

When cancer recurs the most common site is recurrence in the breast or on the chest wall, known as local recurrence. This is not stage 4 disease.

Only when the cancer comes back and affects other parts of the body beyond the breast and axilla such as the bones, lungs, liver and brain is it classed as stage 4 disease. Even when cancer has spread to these sites the cancer is still treatable.

Unusual types of breast cancer
Inflammatory breast cancer
What is inflammatory breast cancer?

An inflammatory breast cancer is one in which the cancer cells produce swelling of the whole breast and cancer cells grow along and block lymph channels in the breast and skin. As a result the breast looks swollen, red and inflamed (this is how the condition gets its name).

Signs and symptoms

The symptoms often develop quite suddenly. The breast may be painful and looks red and inflamed.

The breast feels warm and swollen, and there are often ridges or marks on the skin where the bra presses against the skin. Other symptoms may include a lump or thickening of the breast, discharge from the nipple or a lump underneath the arm.

Treatment

Usually a combination of treatments is needed, including chemotherapy, radiotherapy, hormone therapy and surgery. For most types of breast cancer surgery is usually the first treatment, but for inflammatory breast cancer chemotherapy or radiotherapy is usually given first. Chemotherapy is sometimes combined with trastuzumab if the cancer is HER2 positive (see page 212).

Usually between four and eight doses of chemotherapy are given. The effect of treatment will usually be assessed after four doses of chemotherapy. It is usual to get some reduction in the swelling, redness and tenderness of the breast after chemotherapy is started.

Occasionally the chemotherapy can result in complete disappearance of all cancer at the end of treatment. After chemotherapy the next treatment is usually surgery and/or radiotherapy.

Paget's disease

Paget's disease of the nipple is uncommon. Fewer than five per cent of women with breast cancer have Paget's disease. It can also affect men. In Paget's disease cancer cells grow from the ends of the milk ducts into the skin of the nipple.

The features of Paget's disease are a red scaly nipple. One way in which a doctor can distinguish between Paget's disease and eczema – a chronic skin condition commonly affecting the nipple – is that Paget's disease always affects the nipple first, whereas eczema affects the area around the nipple, known as the areola, first.

Paget's disease also usually affects only one breast whereas eczema often affects both. In Paget's disease the rash can feel itchy and there is often leakage of material from the surface of the nipple.

About half of patients with Paget's disease have an underlying lump. Most patients with cancer and Paget's disease have either DCIS in the ducts underneath the nipple or an invasive cancer somewhere in the breast.

To tell whether an abnormal area on the nipple is Paget's disease, a small biopsy of the skin is taken and sent to the laboratory.

Treatment

If Paget's disease is associated with DCIS or cancer in the underlying breast, treatment is directed at this as described in the next chapter, except that the nipple is always removed.

For Paget's disease that is present on its own, treatment involves surgery to remove the nipple, usually followed by radiotherapy.

Follow-up usually involves annual examination and mammograms.

Lymphoma and sarcoma of the breast

Within the breast there is lymphoid tissue and supporting tissues and occasionally a tumour can develop in these tissues. This is rare. Malignant growths arising in lymphoid tissue are known as lymphomas and malignant growths from fat and fibrous tissue are known as sarcomas.

Metastasis to the breast

Very unusually a cancer at another site, for example a

cancer in the lung or skin, can spread to the breast.
Over 99 per cent of cancers in the breast start in the
breast and are breast cancers. Breast cancers have
particular appearances under the microscope and so, if
your doctor tells you that you have breast cancer, you
can be confident that the growth started in the breast.

KEY POINTS

■ There are several different types of breast cancer, some of which have a better outlook than others

■ Treatment for ductal carcinoma *in situ* (DCIS) should prevent cancer developing; most women with DCIS can be treated by breast-conserving surgery but where DCIS involves a large part of the breast then mastectomy may be needed

■ Important considerations for all breast cancers are whether they have spread to the armpit lymph nodes or to elsewhere in the body

■ Tests are carried out after a breast cancer is diagnosed to check how far the disease has progressed

■ Inflammatory breast cancer, where the breast is red and swollen, is usually treated with chemotherapy first

■ In Paget's disease the nipple is red and scaly. If there is no underlying cancer it is treated by removing the nipple

Treating breast cancer

How is treatment decided?

Once a thorough assessment has been made of the type and extent of disease it is possible to work out the most appropriate treatment for any individual patient. The most important factor determining treatment is the stage of disease.

Treatment may include:

- Surgery

- Radiotherapy

- Hormone therapy

- Chemotherapy

- Biologic therapy.

Often a combination of these treatments is used. Treatment will be chosen depending on what is best for the patient and best for the particular type and stage of cancer. Treatment is decided only after taking into account each individual woman's wishes.

Where there are treatment options these will be explained and the patient invited to share in the treatment decision. If you, as the patient, prefer not to be involved in deciding about treatment then tell your doctor and he or she will advise you as to what he or she thinks is the treatment that is most likely to be effective.

In most cases the first treatment will be surgery followed by radiotherapy to deal with the cancer in the breast and the lymph glands under the arm. This is followed by drug treatment aimed at destroying any undetected cells that may have escaped to other parts of the body.

Breast cancer is a very treatable cancer and is associated with a high cure rate. Treatments for breast cancer are improving and so is survival. Despite the fact that more women are diagnosed with breast cancer every year, the number of women who actually die from breast cancer is falling, which demonstrates how effective current treatments are.

Asking questions and understanding the answers

The shock and stress after a diagnosis of breast cancer can make it hard to think of questions to ask your doctor. It often helps to make a list of questions when you are going to discuss treatment.

To help you remember what the doctor says, there are a number of different options. You may wish to make notes, take a member of your family or a friend with you, or use a tape recorder to record the conversation.

Most breast cancer treatment takes place in specialist breast units, and treatment decisions are usually taken by a team of specialists. You are likely to have different doctors for each type of treatment.

Who looks after me?

The team of doctors involved in your care is likely to include a specialist breast surgeon, and one or more oncologists. Some oncologists specialise in radiotherapy and others in drug treatments such as chemotherapy, hormone therapy or trastuzumab. Yet other oncologists give radiotherapy and drug treatment. When considering treatment other doctors involved include radiologists, who specialise in interpretation of X-rays and scans, and pathologists, who report on the needle biopsies performed when you are first seen at the clinic and the specimens that the surgeons remove. Some breast units have their own plastic surgeons who specialise in managing breast problems, including breast reconstruction. Also involved are breast care nurses who see patients in the clinic to discuss how they are coping with the diagnosis of breast cancer, provide information and act as a link between the patient and the doctors.

Other nurses see patients in clinics (nurse practitioner) and nurses play an enormously important role in research (research nurses) and looking after you while you are in hospital. Diagnostic radiographers take the X-rays, and some also do ultrasound scans; other therapeutic radiographers are involved in giving you radiotherapy. Physiotherapists will give you advice on exercises to stop shoulder stiffness and get you back to normal as soon as possible after any operation. Any team also needs good administrative and secretarial support. There are a huge number of people involved and you may meet some or all of the people listed above during your patient journey.

If you are concerned about whether you are being treated in a specialist unit, ask. If you are unhappy at any stage with your treatment discuss this with your doctors and nurses.

Although very few patients switch to another hospital or request a second opinion, these options are available and you need to be certain that you have confidence in the team of doctors and nurses looking after you.

Treatment generally begins within a few weeks of diagnosis. There is no need to rush to start treatment so there is time for you to talk to your doctors and nurses about it.

All specialist units now have breast care nurses. They will see you after discussion of treatment with your doctor. Patients often find it easier to speak to breast care nurses than they do to doctors. If the treatment plan that you receive is not clear, ask the breast care nurse.

Many units give patients a treatment diary, which is helpful because it allows you to write down which treatments you are likely to get and the exact dates of any appointments or operations.

What types of treatment are there?

Treatment of cancer consists of:

- local therapies (which treat the breast and armpit)

- systemic therapies (which treat any cells that could have escaped anywhere else in the body).

Local therapies

Surgery and radiotherapy are local treatments. They remove or destroy cancer cells in the breast and the lymph glands.

Systemic therapies

Hormone therapy, chemotherapy and biologic therapy are systemic therapies. They enter the bloodstream and destroy or control cancer throughout the body.

Some women with breast cancer will have systemic therapy as their initial treatment. This may be given to shrink the tumour before surgery or radiotherapy either to make surgery possible if it is not an option or to allow less extensive surgery.

Most women who have surgery and radiotherapy will have systemic treatment after their local treatment. Other women whose cancer has spread may only have systemic treatments so cancer cells at these sites are destroyed or controlled.

How do I find out more about treatment?

Most women want to know how treatment will change their lives and how they will look during and after treatment. Doctors and nurses are the best people to describe each treatment, the side effects and the expected results of treatment.

Breast care nurses usually have pictures of patients who have had different surgical treatments. They can also arrange for you to meet women who have had each type of treatment.

As well as getting information from your doctors and nurses, you can get information from a number of self-help groups. They have telephone lines that you can call. This allows you either to speak to someone or to get information sent to you through the post. You can also get lots of information from their websites.

The most commonly used organisations are Breast Cancer Care, Breakthrough Breast Cancer and Macmillan Cancer Relief. Their contact details are included in 'Further information' (see page 220).

Your role in treatment

Where there are choices or options for treatment these will be explained to you. If you have concerns or preferences make sure that your breast care nurse and your doctors are aware of these. Treatment involves a partnership of you, your doctors, nurses and other members of the breast cancer team.

Complementary medicine

Most doctors are concerned at any stage of disease if women with breast cancer opt solely for alternative or complementary medicine when their disease can be effectively treated by conventional medical treatments. Nevertheless, many people find great comfort in having some input into the control of their condition by visiting herbalists or other practitioners of so-called natural medicines.

The commonsense approach is to discuss this openly and honestly with your doctor. He or she is unlikely to raise any objections, provided that you do not opt for complementary medicine instead of conventional treatment.

KEY POINTS

■ Following a thorough assessment an appropriate treatment can be worked out

■ The most important factor determining treatment is the stage of the disease

■ Treatment is decided only after taking account of each individual woman's wishes

■ Breast cancer is a very treatable cancer and associated with a high cure rate

■ Make a list of questions when going to discuss treatment

■ Consider taking a friend or relative with you when going to discuss treatment

Surgery for breast cancer

This is the most common treatment used for women with breast cancer. There are several different types of surgery.

When the cancer is relatively small, under three centimetres in size, it is usually possible for the surgeon to remove the lump along with a small amount of surrounding normal breast tissue; this is called breast-conserving surgery. This is usually combined with removal of some or all the lymph nodes under the arm. If the cancer is larger, or affects more than one area of the breast, or if the woman prefers, the whole breast is removed, this operation being known as mastectomy.

Other options for larger cancers are the use of drugs to shrink the cancer or more complex surgery, usually involving a plastic or oncoplastic surgeon to remove the cancer but leave the breast shape intact.

Breast-conserving surgery

This is also known as wide local excision (or lumpectomy). The aim of breast-conserving surgery is to remove the tumour with a clear rim of normal tissue around it. If all the cancer is not removed, there is a high chance that the cancer will re-grow. Radiotherapy is almost always given to the breast after breast-conserving surgery.

Margins

Margins, also known as 'margins of resection', refer to the distance between a tumour and the edge of the surrounding tissue that is removed along with it.

When a tumour is removed, some tissue surrounding it is also removed by a lumpectomy. The tumour with surrounding tissue is rolled in a special ink so that the outer edges, or margins, are clearly visible under a microscope. A pathologist checks the tissue under a microscope to see if the margins are free of cancer cells.

Depending upon what the pathologist sees, the margins of a tumour are described as follows:

- Positive margins: cancer cells extend out to the edge or are very close to the edge of the tissue removed by the surgeon

- Negative margins: no cancer cells are found at the inked margin and there is a thin rim of normal tissue, indicating that the cancer has been completely removed.

Knowing how close cancer cells are to the edge of the removed tissue helps in making the right treatment decisions. This is especially important in deciding whether additional surgery is needed.

Breast-conserving surgery

Breast-conserving surgery ranges from lumpectomy or wide local excision (in which the tumour is removed with a small amount of surrounding tissue, sometimes referred to as a margin), to quadrantectomy in which about a quarter of the breast is removed.

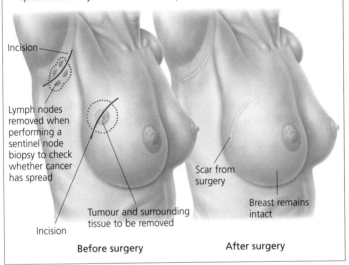

Incision

Lymph nodes removed when performing a sentinel node biopsy to check whether cancer has spread

Incision

Tumour and surrounding tissue to be removed

Scar from surgery

Breast remains intact

Before surgery

After surgery

Patients who are suitable for breast-conserving surgery are patients who have:

- a single cancer in the breast that measures three centimetres or less

- no evidence of spread beyond the lymph glands under the arm

- a breast size sufficient to produce a good cosmetic result after removal of the cancer.

Patients who are not usually considered for breast-conserving surgery are:

- those in whom cancer is locally advanced or the lymph nodes are stuck to each other

- those in whom cancer has spread beyond the breast and lymph glands

- women who prefer a mastectomy

- where removal of the cancer will leave a distorted breast.

There are some other reasons why a patient is sometimes not considered for breast-conserving surgery:

- If the tumour is in the central part of the breast, although it is usually possible to remove the nipple and still leave a reasonable result, results from this type of surgery do not always produce a satisfactory result so mastectomy is sometimes advised.

- Patients with specific diseases such as certain collagen vascular diseases, including systemic lupus erythematosus and polyarteritis nodosa, may not be suitable for radiotherapy which is usually given after breast-conserving surgery so mastectomy is usually advised for such patients.

- Where there is more than one tumour in the breast: until recently most women with more than one cancer in the breast were treated by mastectomy but there is good evidence that, provided that both cancers can be removed to clear margins, breast-conserving surgery is possible.

- Women with a strong family history of breast cancer or women who are carrying BRCA-1 or

BRCA-2 mutations should have a thorough discussion of the pros and cons of lumpectomy as they have a higher risk of the cancer returning than women who do not carry an abnormal gene.

The balance between tumour size (assessed by imaging such as ultrasound) and the volume of the woman's breast is the main factor that determines whether a patient is suitable for a lumpectomy. If a patient has a large breast, it may be possible to remove a cancer of larger than three centimetres by breast-conserving surgery. In contrast, in a patient with small breasts removing a two-centimetre cancer may produce an unsatisfactory breast shape after surgery. Tumour size does not relate to the chances of the cancer returning in the breast.

Although most surgeons perform lumpectomies or wide excisions, some surgeons remove larger portions of tissue and do an operation called a quadrantectomy.

It is possible to remove about ten per cent of the breast volume without leaving a deformed breast. If you are having breast-conserving surgery, ask your surgeon what operation will be performed and how your breast is likely to look after surgery.

A wide local excision involves making an incision (cut) in the skin over the breast cancer and removing the cancer with a rim of surrounding breast tissue. After removal of the cancer, any bleeding is stopped and the skin is closed with an invisible stitch, which does not need to be removed.

If the cancer cannot be felt by the surgeon, it will be marked for the surgeon by a radiologist or radiographer in the X-ray department so that it can be removed. Methods available for marking cancers are described in the section on needle localisation biopsy (page 56).

While you are unconscious the surgeon will usually take an X-ray of the area removed to make sure that all the abnormality seen on the original mammogram has been removed. If the X-ray shows that the area of abnormality is close to one of the edges, the surgeon will remove more tissue from this area before stitching the wound.

Problems that can happen after wide local excision

The most common complications immediately after operation are bleeding and feeling unwell after a general anaesthetic (see below).

As a result of removal of the cancer with some surrounding tissue, the treated breast may be smaller than the normal breast after surgery. Depending on the position of the tumour, the treated breast may also change in shape.

About one in ten women gets an unsatisfactory cosmetic result after wide excision and radiotherapy. In these women, it is often possible to reshape the breast at a later date.

Breast-conserving surgery is successful at removal of the cancer and all the surrounding abnormal area in between 80 and 85 women out of 100. In between 15 and 20, when the cancer is looked at under the microscope, the pathologist reports that there is either invasive cancer or more often ductal carcinoma *in situ* (DCIS) at or close to one edge of the tissue removed, that is the margins are positive or involved.

The problem is that the surgeon cannot feel the DCIS when he or she is operating. Just because the surgeon has not removed all the cancer or DCIS does not mean that he or she is a bad surgeon; it is just that this type of disease cannot be felt by the surgeon.

If you are in that 15 to 20 per cent whose cancer has not been removed at one operation you will need a second operation to remove any remaining invasive cancer or DCIS in your breast. This usually means further removal of breast tissue known as a re-excision, although sometimes the pathologist reports that the cancer extends to many of the edges or margins of the tissue removed and a mastectomy may be required to clear all the disease.

Even if the pathologist reports that all the cancer cells have been removed, breast-conserving surgery is almost always followed by radiotherapy. The radiotherapy treats the remaining breast tissue and makes sure that any abnormal cells that could have been left behind elsewhere in the breast are destroyed by it.

The chances of survival are exactly the same whether a woman is treated by breast-conserving surgery (lumpectomy) and radiotherapy or mastectomy. Many women think that mastectomy is safer, but it is not necessarily.

The advantages of having a lumpectomy include that you still have your breast, which makes it easier when you wear clothes. It may also mean that you may feel more confident and women tend to report fewer sexual problems after lumpectomy than after mastectomy.

Many women are given the choice by the surgeon whether to have a lumpectomy and radiotherapy or mastectomy. It is important that you discuss this issue with your partner, surgeon and breast care nurse and, if you feel it appropriate, your GP.

If your surgeon gives you this option, it means that he or she is very confident that breast-conserving surgery will be successful in your case. In this situation, talking to somebody who has had the different operations can be helpful. Take your time before deciding and if you cannot decide tell your doctor.

Mastectomy

Between one in three and one in four women who have surgery for breast cancer cannot have breast-conserving surgery. Some women prefer mastectomy either because it may avoid radiotherapy or because they feel more secure with mastectomy than breast-conserving surgery.

There is no advantage to having your breast removed if it does not need to be removed. If your initial instinct is that you wish to choose a mastectomy, think about it carefully. When some women realise that mastectomy is not going to improve their outcome, women who otherwise would have chosen mastectomy change their mind and decide to keep the breast.

There are situations where a woman with a lump smaller than three centimetres may be advised to have a mastectomy. The following are the main ones:

● If there is more than one lump in the breast. Early research suggested that, if all the individual lumps were removed, there was a slightly greater chance that cancerous lumps were quite likely to develop later in other parts of the same breast. More recent work has suggested that it is safe to do two lumpectomies, provided that clear margins are obtained round both cancers. It depends on where the lumps are in the breast; if the two cancers are close to each other it may be easy to remove them and give radiotherapy and save the breast. If the two lumps are widely separated, it depends on whether the lumps can be removed and leave enough breast tissue to leave the breast shape intact.

- The cancer is directly under the nipple, so that the nipple would have to be removed at the same time. Rather than leave the breast without a nipple, it is sometimes, although not in most women, better to remove the breast altogether and consider a breast reconstruction (see page 177).

- Sometimes an operation to remove the lump is not successful, because the cancer or the DCIS is more extensive than was evident on X-rays. A second operation to remove more tissue can solve the problem, but if there is widespread change it is usual to remove the whole breast to ensure that no disease is left behind.

- Tissue surrounding an invasive cancer is affected by a large area of DCIS (this is usually visible on the mammogram). If all the disease cannot be removed by lumpectomy, a mastectomy may be the safest option.

- Where removal of the lump would result in a grossly misshapen breast, for instance in a woman with a lump between two and three centimetres in a smaller breast.

Mastectomy is an operation that removes the breast tissue. There are different types of mastectomy. Women who have mastectomy can also choose either to have or not to have a breast reconstruction. This is considered later, on page 177.

Different types of mastectomy

Simple mastectomy

A simple mastectomy removes the breast tissue but does not remove all the lymph glands or the chest wall muscles. If you have larger breasts then it may be better to remove the breast through the type of cut used for breast reduction which gives an upside-down T scar.

When performing a mastectomy a cut is made above and below the nipple and all the breast tissue down to the chest wall muscle is removed. Sufficient skin is removed so that at the end of the operation there will be no loose skin and a flat straight scar is left on the chest wall. The exact direction of the wound scar depends on where the tumour is situated but most mastectomy scars are horizontal or diagonal.

Modified radical mastectomy

This is performed through the same incision as a simple mastectomy. It involves removal of the breast and all the lymph nodes that drain the breast in the axilla. It is usually possible to do this without causing any damage to the chest wall muscles.

Radical mastectomy

This operation is hardly ever performed any more and involves removal of the breast, the axillary nodes and the underlying chest wall muscles.

Subcutaneous mastectomy

This is an operation that is performed in women with smaller cancers or DCIS, or who are at high risk of

Simple mastectomy

Simple mastectomy is the surgical removal of one or both breasts and is often combined with removal of a few of the lymph nodes under the arm. Breast-sparing techniques may be used to preserve the patient's breast skin and nipple, which is helpful in cosmetic breast reconstruction.

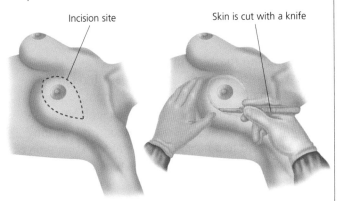

Incision site

Skin is cut with a knife

1. The incision site is marked on the suface of the skin

2. The skin is incised in the area to be removed

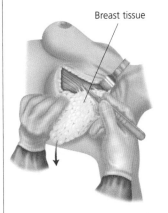

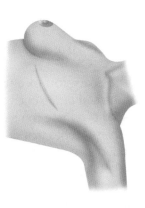

Breast tissue

3. The incision is deepened and all the breast tissue removed

4. After thorough cleaning by irrigation the wound is closed

breast cancer. It removes all the breast tissue, but keeps as much skin as possible so that, when the breast is reconstructed, it looks as similar to the original breast shape as possible with very few visible scars. This operation is performed through an incision either under the nipple or at the edge of the breast. The nipple and the areola are left intact and no skin is removed.

Skin-sparing mastectomy

It is also possible to remove the breast through an incision that removes only a small amount of skin either over the cancer or around the nipple area. The advantage of a skin-sparing mastectomy is that the scars are kept to a minimum while at the same time all the breast tissue and skin over the tumour or the nipple are removed.

Removal of lymph glands during mastectomy

If all the lymph glands are being removed (axillary node clearance) or some of the axillary lymph glands are being removed (sentinel node biopsy or axillary node sample), this is usually performed through the same cut (incision) used to remove the breast.

What can you expect after the operation?

At the end of the operation, one or two drains are placed and these come out below the wound. Drains are plastic tubes that drain fluid which the body produces into the space under the skin. These drains are left in place for between three and five days. They are removed when the amount of fluid coming out of the drain reduces.

After mastectomy you may be in hospital between one and seven days depending on the extent of the surgery, whether you had a reconstruction at the same time and the policy of the hospital at which you are treated.

Problems that can occur after mastectomy

The most common complications immediately after operation are bleeding and feeling unwell after a general anaesthetic.

The edges of the mastectomy wound may not heal because of problems with the blood supply. If this happens the edges may become inflamed and can scab. This usually settles without any specific treatment. It is more likely when more skin is kept as in a subcutaneous (or skin-sparing) mastectomy and is also more common in women with diabetes or who smoke.

There can be extra tissue or lumpiness at the outer edge of the scar under the armpit. This lumpiness and swelling can settle over a period of time. Occasionally this extra tissue (the common name for this is a 'dog ear') needs to be trimmed at a later date.

Fluid can build up after the drains are removed which causes a swelling under the wound, called a seroma. If this is uncomfortable then a needle can be used to drain it.

Looking at yourself either from above or in the mirror after surgery can be difficult, traumatic and very emotional. Some women are surprised at how neat the scar is, but most find it upsetting when they see it for the first time. There is no right time to look. Some women prefer to wait; others want to look immediately. You might want to do this when you have someone with you such as a breast care nurse.

Options for women with large tumours

If your surgeon tells you that your tumour is not suitable for breast-conserving surgery, there may be other options for you, which might include one of the following.

Primary systemic therapy

This involves having drug therapy as the first treatment – so-called primary systemic therapy. The aim of this treatment is to shrink the cancer down to a size where it can be removed by a lumpectomy. The drug treatment is most commonly chemotherapy, but increasingly hormone therapy is being used to shrink cancers in older women.

Very wide excision with reconstruction

Removal of a large part of the breast and replacement with tissue from elsewhere in the body (usually the back) is an option for some women. This is called partial breast reconstruction (see page 179).

Mammoplasty

If removal of the cancer would make the breast smaller, it is possible at the same time to make the other breast smaller to match. This type of surgery is known as reduction mammoplasty. It is performed in only a few units, and is suitable for women with large tumours in reasonable sized breasts. If you have larger breasts and have always wanted them to be made smaller this may be an option for you.

Axillary surgical treatment for breast cancer

One of the first places that breast cancer spreads to is

the lymph glands under the arm. There are a number of different axillary lymph node operations that are performed and the choice of surgery depends on the chances that the lymph nodes are likely to be affected.

Sometimes it is possible to see abnormal lymph nodes before operation using ultrasound and to biopsy them. In most instances, however, it is necessary for the surgeon to remove some or all of the lymph glands to have them tested.

When you have either breast-conserving surgery or mastectomy the surgeon will usually check whether your lymph glands are involved by removing a sample of them or all the lymph glands under your arm if they have been tested and shown to be affected.

Lymph node biopsy

A lymph node biopsy removes lymph node tissue with a needle to be looked at under a microscope for signs of infection or a disease, such as cancer. The needle can be a fine needle or a core needle (see page 53).

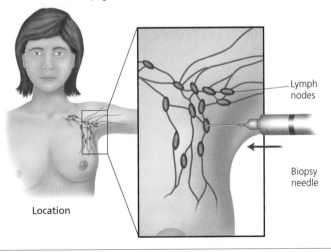

Lymph nodes

Biopsy needle

Location

There are around 20 lymph glands under your arm and these are the most common place to which breast cancer may spread. Knowing whether this has happened and how many lymph glands are affected is important in both assessing the stage of the cancer and deciding the best type of treatment.

If all the surgeon wants to do is to test the lymph glands, removing the few lymph glands that drain the cancer is sufficient. If the lymph glands are known to be affected, removing them is effective treatment at controlling any disease in these lymph glands. To know exactly how many lymph glands are involved it is necessary to remove all of them. You do not need the lymph glands under your arm and your body can manage to function perfectly normally without these. Removing all the glands does, however, increase the rate of postoperative complications and increases the long-term chances of you getting swelling of your arm (lymphoedema – see page 121).

Sampling the glands to test them

There are now a variety of methods available to check whether breast cancer has spread into the lymph glands.

Sentinel node biopsy

The first lymph node(s) draining a cancer is known as the sentinel node(s). In sentinel node biopsy a specially trained surgeon removes only these sentinel nodes to see if the cancer has reached them.

The sentinel nodes are identified by injecting blue dye plus a radioactive tracer material into the breast. This passes up to the lymph glands, and the surgeon then finds the draining or sentinel lymph glands because they are either stained blue or radioactive.

The radioactivity is detected with a small hand-held probe, which makes a loud noise when a lot of radioactivity is present in a particular lymph node. On average, a surgeon will find three sentinel nodes per patient.

Usually the radioactive injection is given two to three hours before surgery. The blue dye is injected at the time of surgery after you are unconscious. It has recently been shown that injecting both the radiotracer and blue dye together just before operation when you are under anaesthetic produces satisfactory results and saves the patient from having an injection when they are awake.

The most common places for injecting the blue dye and the radioactivity are around the cancer, into the skin over the cancer and underneath the nipple. Wherever the breast is injected, drainage is to the same few lymph nodes under the arm.

Sentinel node biopsy is successful at finding nodes in 98 of every 100 women. If the surgeon is planning a sentinel node biopsy but no sentinel nodes are found he or she will perform an axillary sample or remove sufficient nodes to check whether the cancer has reached them.

If a sentinel node biopsy shows that your lymph glands are affected by cancer your doctor may recommend that you have either a second operation to remove all the remaining lymph glands or radiotherapy to the remaining glands.

Axillary node sampling
Lymph node sampling aims to remove four lymph glands to check whether any of them is affected by cancer. Any cancer that spreads to the lymph glands

Sentinel node biopsy

This is a minimally invasive procedure in which lymph nodes that drain the site of a cancerous tumour are first identified as sentinel nodes and then removed for microscopic analysis. The lymph node(s) closest to a tumour serve to filter and trap cancer cells. These nodes are known as sentinel nodes because they act like sentries and warn doctors that a patient's cancer has spread.

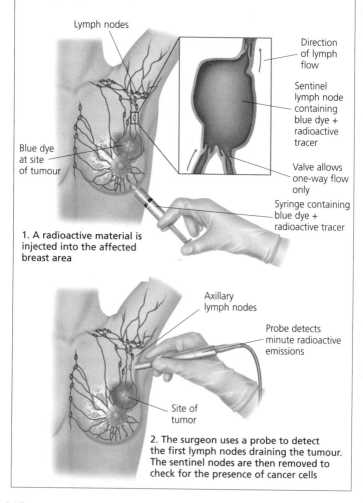

Lymph nodes

Direction of lymph flow

Sentinel lymph node containing blue dye + radioactive tracer

Valve allows one-way flow only

Syringe containing blue dye + radioactive tracer

Blue dye at site of tumour

1. A radioactive material is injected into the affected breast area

Axillary lymph nodes

Probe detects minute radioactive emissions

Site of tumor

2. The surgeon uses a probe to detect the first lymph nodes draining the tumour. The sentinel nodes are then removed to check for the presence of cancer cells

under your arm affects the lowest lymph glands first, which is why sampling four of these low lymph glands checks, with a great degree of accuracy, whether any glands are affected.

Sampling is usually combined with injection of blue dye under the nipple to increase the certainty that the nodes removed are likely to induce the sentinel nodes draining the cancer.

Both sentinel node biopsy and axillary node sampling are performed through a small cut (incision) in your armpit just below where the hair grows. At the end of the operation the wound is closed with an invisible stitch that does not need to be removed.

If any of the sentinel nodes or sampled nodes contain cancer, the remaining lymph glands will need to be treated either by a second operation to remove the remaining nodes or by a course of radiotherapy.

Selection of different axillary treatments

Sentinel lymph node biopsy is a good option when there are no obvious lymph glands to feel and no abnormal lymph glands visible on ultrasound. It can be used before or after chemotherapy.

Most units have a policy on who is suitable for sentinel node biopsy. It is important to understand exactly which operation you are having and why the surgeon is recommencing that particular procedure for you. Not all breast units offer sentinel node biopsy. Ask because it may be possible to refer you to another hospital if that is the best option for you.

Axillary node clearance

Lymph node clearance aims to remove all the lymph glands. It checks exactly how many are involved. It removes all the nodes so that no affected nodes are left behind. It is performed only in patients whose lymph glands have been shown to be affected by scanning and biopsy of the nodes either with a needle or after surgery to remove the sentinel nodes.

The operation is performed through a slightly larger cut in your armpit than that used for sentinel node biopsy. At the end of the operation the wound is closed with an invisible stitch that does not need to be removed.

A drain is usually placed after axillary clearance to remove the fluid that the body produces in the days after the operation. The drain usually remains in place for between three and five days. It is possible for you to go home with your drain still in place. Please ask your surgeon if you would like further information about this.

Problems that can happen after axillary node surgery

The most common problem is pain, swelling and discomfort under the arm which lasts for a few weeks. Do not be afraid to take regular painkillers. Ensure that the arm keeps mobile by practising the exercises taught to you while in the ward.

The most common complications immediately after operation are bleeding and feeling unwell after a general anaesthetic.

Numbness

There are a number of nerves that pass through the armpit to the inner side of the arm. The nerves that supply feeling to the upper inner part of the arm are sometimes damaged during removal of all the lymph glands. Your surgeon will make every attempt not to damage these nerves. They are much less commonly damaged during sentinel lymph node biopsy.

Even if the nerves have not been cut they will be stretched and so this area may feel numb and it will take some time after surgery before normal feeling returns. You should therefore be prepared for some slight loss of feeling in the upper inner part of the arm on the side of the surgery. In about half of patients this recovers during the first few months after operation.

Shoulder stiffness

You will be taught a series of exercises after surgery by a physiotherapist. It is important that these are carried out. Shoulder stiffness and reduction in the movement of the shoulder are common problems in those who do not manage to do their shoulder exercises.

You may get some pain and discomfort after surgery and experience soreness when performing your exercises. Do not be afraid to take regular painkillers after surgery because this will make it less painful and allow you to do your exercises with less discomfort.

During this period of recovery, there may be some pain or discomfort down the inside of your upper arm, but this usually settles after a few weeks.

Lymphoedema

Lymphoedema or swelling of the arm (caused by collection of fluid in the tissues after removal of or damage to lymph nodes) can follow removal of all the axillary lymph nodes (axillary clearance) or may occur if, after a sentinel node biopsy or axillary node sampling, radiotherapy is given to the axilla.

About 6 in every 100 women develop significant arm swelling after axillary clearance. The severity of swelling and chances of getting swelling are much less after sentinel node biopsy and radiotherapy.

Arm swelling or lymphoedema can occur many years after an operation. Specialist assessment and treatment are required and may involve referral to a physiotherapist.

Treatment consists of skin care, regular massage, active exercise, and wearing a sleeve or other compression garment.

Physical management of lymphoedema

Lymphoedema is chronic swelling that is essentially incurable. Physical symptoms can be controlled with treatment.

The four cornerstones of treatment are:

1. **Skin care** to maintain good skin condition and reduce the risk of infection

2. **Exercise** to promote lymph flow and maintain good limb function

3. **Manual lymphatic drainage** – gentle skin massage encourages lymph flow and is carried out by a trained therapist

4. **Support/compression** – multilayer lymphoedema bandaging is applied to reduce the size and improve the condition of the limb to allow fitting of elastic compression garments, which, when fitted correctly, control swelling and encourage lymph flow

General complications after surgery for breast cancer
Bleeding

Even though all visible bleeding is stopped during the operation, bleeding from the cut edges of the breast tissue can occasionally start afterwards and cause blood to collect in the wound. This is uncommon, and happens in 1–2 of every 100 patients. It is more common after mastectomy than lumpectomy.

The normal time for this to develop is within the first few hours after the operation. This is the reason for checking the wound after surgery. If a large amount of blood collects (called a haematoma), this needs to be drained, usually by a second operation.

Seroma

The body produces its own natural healing fluid. Some people produce more than others and this can cause swelling at the site where the lump or the lymph glands have been removed. This is known as a seroma.

The fluid may require removal with a needle and syringe when you return to the clinic. As the area is often numb after surgery, this is usually a painless procedure.

Infection

Any operation wound can become infected. It is uncommon to get infection in breast wounds but approximately 1 in 10 women does get some infection after breast cancer surgery. If infection develops, it is often a week after surgery before any features show.

Signs of wound infection include the wound being red, swollen and very tender, and there may also be a discharge through the wound. Most infections settle with antibiotics.

Deep venous thrombosis

This is when clots form in the veins of the legs. These clots can move from the veins in the legs up to the lung (called a pulmonary embolus). This is uncommon because, when you are in hospital, the doctors and nurses take specific precautions to stop this happening.

These precautions involve wearing stockings to support the veins, having regular injections into your stomach of drugs that thin the blood to stop it clotting, and having special boots that you wear in the operating theatre which keep the blood in your legs flowing.

Pain after operation

Although the acute pain after surgery will settle within a few weeks of the operation, the area where you have had surgery can feel uncomfortable for months and years.

After breast surgery, some women develop chronic pain. This can be made worse if you suddenly increase activity such as going to the gym or gardening. Pain is rarely a symptom that the cancer is back and usually responds to medication and regular gentle exercise.

Frozen shoulder

This is not uncommon after an operation on the lymph glands under the arm. It is easier to stop this than treat it. Following the exercises recommended by your care team usually prevents this complication. If you find your shoulder becoming stiff and your shoulder movement is restricted report this to your doctor.

Fat necrosis

Any operation damages the surrounding tissue. This is sometimes a problem for the blood supply of the fat in the breast (or in tissue brought into the breast for a reconstruction). This can cause areas of fat to die (necrosis) which can form a worrying lump. Simple tests can quickly prove that such a lump is innocent.

Cording

After surgery on the breast or axilla, blood and lymphatic vessels in the area, including in the upper arm, get blocked or are no longer connected to a lymph node, so the vessel collapses and becomes fibrous. If the fibrous tissue tightens it produces tight bands across the armpit, below the breast and down the arm. This is colloquially called 'cording'. It can be painful. Regular exercises stretch the cords and they usually settle with time. Rarely the cords need to be divided surgically.

KEY POINTS

- Surgery for breast cancer usually involves either an operation to remove the cancer lump (followed by radiotherapy – called breast-conserving surgery) or an operation to remove the whole breast (called mastectomy)

- The decision on the appropriate surgery depends on the site and the size of the cancer in the breast relative to the size of the breast

- If an invasive cancer is present the armpit lymph nodes will be checked to see if there is any sign of spread of the cancer

- This is best done by taking the first few lymph nodes that drain the cancer (sentinel node biopsy)

- Axillary node clearance is a bigger operation which removes all the nodes in the armpit if there are cancer cells in the lymph nodes

- If only a few lymph nodes have been taken and there are cancer cells in them, further treatment with either another operation to remove the rest of the lymph nodes or radiotherapy to the armpit will be needed

Radiotherapy treatment for breast cancer

How does radiotherapy work?

Radiotherapy kills cells by using X-rays to damage the cells in the body that are growing. Fortunately in the normal breast only a few cells are growing at any one time whereas in a cancer there are many more growing cells so radiotherapy produces much more damage to the cancer cells than the normal tissue. Radiotherapy is used frequently after women have had breast surgery.

Radiotherapy can be given:

- after breast-conserving surgery because it has been shown that it dramatically reduces the chances of cancer returning

- after mastectomy, but it tends to be restricted to women in whom the chances of the cancer returning without radiotherapy are significant

- to the lymph glands under the arm if only some of the lymph glands have been removed and these are affected by cancer

- to control some cancers not suitable for surgery, for example it can dry up cancers that are bleeding

- to shrink cancers before an operation

- to treat cancers that recur or spread to other parts of the body (bones or brain)

- to the lymph nodes in the lower neck (supraclavicular region) and to the nodes behind the breast bone known as the internal mammary nodes if these are affected or are at risk of being affected.

Who gets radiotherapy after mastectomy?

Studies have shown that radiotherapy after mastectomy in some women not only reduces the chances of the cancer returning but also improves survival. If you have a large cancer or involved nodes, or the cancer is very close to the back of the breast making it more difficult for the surgeon to get a good clear margin, you are more likely to receive radiotherapy after mastectomy. Trials are ongoing to try to identify exactly who benefits and, more importantly, who can safely avoid radiotherapy. After mastectomy radiotherapy can be given to the chest wall, under where the breast was, to the nodes alongside the breastbone (internal mammary nodes) and to the nodes in the axilla and supraclavicular region.

Side effects

There are relatively few side effects from radiotherapy. You may find that you become tired more easily. A few days after starting radiotherapy you may also find that your skin looks red and feels a little sore, rather like you have spent too much time in the sun.

Towards the end of treatment you can also get some bleeding from the treated skin. As with sunburned skin, your skin can feel sore when you put water on it. Generally radiotherapists prefer women to keep the treated area dry and apply local creams.

You should follow the advice given by your own radiotherapist as to how your skin is managed. You need to make sure that you are careful about not exposing radiotherapy-treated skin to the sun. If you do, you need to use sun block.

Some patients who have radiotherapy after breast surgery or to treat a breast cancer do get a slight cough. This is caused by the fact that when radiotherapy is given to the breast a small part of the lung underneath the breast also receives some of the radiotherapy dose. This can cause slight scarring in the lung, which results in irritation and development of a cough.

Very occasionally you can also become breathless. There are good treatments for this so, if you experience these problems, discuss with your doctor. These symptoms usually settle quickly when suitable treatment is started.

How is radiotherapy given?

Radiotherapy is a course of treatment given in the hospital radiotherapy department. It is usually given daily from Monday to Friday and lasts between three and six weeks.

Most radiotherapy is given as external radiotherapy. This means that nothing is in contact with your skin. Another option is to give internal radiotherapy by placing wires or a balloon containing radioactive

Radiotherapy

Radiotherapy is a cancer treatment that uses targeted radiation to kill cancer cells. It is usually given as a series of short, daily sessions from Monday to Friday, with a rest at the weekend.

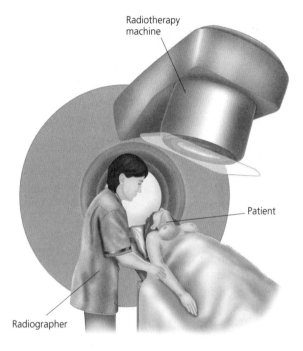

Radiotherapy machine

Patient

Radiographer

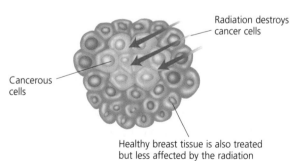

Radiation destroys cancer cells

Cancerous cells

Healthy breast tissue is also treated but less affected by the radiation

substances into the breast. These wires and balloons are placed under general anaesthetic.

It is possible to give radiotherapy during surgery – known as intraoperative radiotherapy. A balloon or device can also be placed in the breast to deliver radiotherapy to a part of the breast after surgery. These types of local radiotherapy are currently undergoing trials. The results so far look promising, but it will be necessary to wait some years to find out if they are safe in the long term.

Planning your treatment

Your first visit to the radiotherapy department will be a planning visit. You will be asked to lie under a machine called a simulator which then takes X-rays and scans of the area that is going to be treated. Planning usually includes a CT scan, so the exact doses and direction of the beams to be used can be worked out.

These scans and X-rays allow the doctors to work out exactly how the treatment should be delivered. Often marks will be placed on your skin to help the radiographer who gives the treatment to position you accurately when you attend for your radiotherapy.

If you are having radiotherapy to the breast you will need to have good movement of your shoulder and arm. If the movement of your shoulder is limited it is important to inform your doctors so that you can get some help from a physiotherapist to improve the range of movement so radiotherapy can be given effectively.

As well as a standard dose of radiotherapy, women who have had a lumpectomy may also be given an extra dose to the localised area around where the cancer was situated in the breast. This is known as a boost.

This extra dose appears to be more important in younger rather than older women and significantly reduces the chances that the cancer will return in the breast. The boost is usually given as an extra few days at the end of treatment using the radiotherapy machine but it can also be given by placing wires in the breast – called interstitial radiotherapy.

KEY POINTS

- Radiotherapy is usually given to the breast after a breast cancer lump has been removed

- Radiotherapy is sometimes given after mastectomy to the remaining tissue on the chest and to the lymph nodes in the armpit or neck if they are involved with cancer

- A course of radiotherapy usually lasts from three to six weeks

Drug treatment (systemic therapy)

When are drugs used?

Surgery alone was used to treat breast cancer until it became clear that some cancers had spread to other parts of the body by the time surgery was performed. After such surgery, untreated cancer cells grew in the parts of the body that they had spread to and this caused symptoms and problems in these areas.

Studies have now shown that women with early breast cancer who receive drug treatment or systemic therapy after surgery to treat cells that have spread have a better outcome, with a longer survival and fewer recurrences.

Drug treatments in common usage for breast cancer include:

- hormone therapy

- chemotherapy

- newer targeted biologic treatments such as trastuzumab.

The same drugs are used to shrink cancers before surgery (sometimes called neoadjuvant therapy), after surgery as adjuvant therapy (treatment given in addition to surgery and radiotherapy) and to treat breast cancer that has returned or spread.

Choosing treatments for individual patients is not straightforward. It is usually a balance of weighing up the benefits compared with the side effects. When deciding on a particular treatment the following factors need to be considered:

- the risk of the cancer returning

- the likely benefits of the treatment

- the risks and side effects of the treatment

- the general health of the patient

- the views of the patient.

Hormone therapies
Why is oestrogen important?

The hormones oestrogen and progesterone play an important part in the control of growth and development of the normal breast. At puberty these hormones increase in amount and are responsible for the development of the breast. During pregnancy as hormone levels increase, growth of breast tissue allows production of milk.

As well as controlling the activity of normal cells, oestrogen is also involved in controlling the activity of cancer cells. About three-quarters of breast cancers contain receptors for oestrogen and/or progesterone within the cells.

Many breast cancers are dependent on oestrogen and progesterone for their growth and removal of oestrogen can stop cancer cells growing and cause them to die.

It is now routine to test breast cancers for oestrogen receptors (ERs, where E is for estrogen – the American spelling) and progesterone receptors (PgRs) (see page 81). Some tumours do not have any oestrogen receptors and are referred to as ER negative and therefore not dependent on hormones.

Both premenopausal and postmenopausal women produce oestrogen. In premenopausal women the major source of oestrogen is the ovaries. The brain controls the amount of oestrogen that the ovaries produce by producing a hormone called luteinising hormone-releasing hormone (LHRH).

The LHRH stimulates a gland under the brain, known as the pituitary gland, to produce hormones that then stimulate the ovaries to produce oestrogen.

In postmenopausal women male hormones, which are produced from a gland that sits on the kidneys, called the adrenal gland, are converted to oestrogen in fat, muscle, liver, breast tissue and even within breast cancers.

The conversion from male to female hormones is through an enzyme called aromatase. There are now very specific drugs that block this enzyme and they are called aromatase inhibitors.

How do hormone treatments work?
Hormonal treatments work by either:

The female reproductive organs

This shows a cross-section through the female reproductive organs. Your uterus or womb is the size and shape of an upside-down pear. It is a muscle with a central cavity connected to the outside by the vagina. It is also connected to the ovaries by two fallopian tubes.

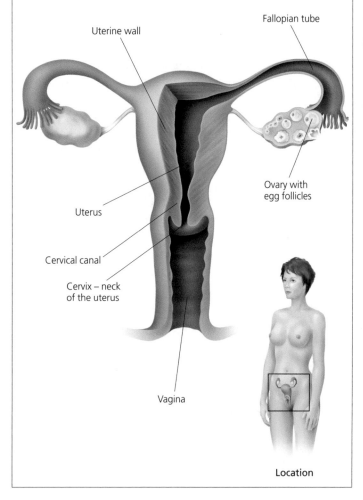

Uterine wall

Fallopian tube

Ovary with egg follicles

Uterus

Cervical canal

Cervix – neck of the uterus

Vagina

Location

- blocking the action of oestrogen or

- preventing the production of oestrogen.

These treatments are very effective and generally produce fewer side effects when compared with chemotherapy. Women whose tumours are ER negative do not benefit from these treatments.

As well as reducing the risk of cancer returning, these drugs are also effective at reducing the development of new breast cancers. There are a variety of hormone treatments including:

- removal of the ovaries

- suppression of the ovaries

to reduce oestrogen production in premenopausal women.

Removal of the ovaries

The ovaries can be removed by an operation (oophorectomy) or radiotherapy can be given to the ovaries, which stops them functioning. The easiest way of removing the ovaries is via keyhole surgery using a laparoscope. The problem with surgical oophorectomy is that it produces a permanent and rapid onset of menopausal symptoms.

Nevertheless it is effective and is particularly important for women who have *BRCA*-1 or *BRCA*-2 gene mutations who are at increased risk of breast and ovarian cancer. Removal of the ovaries in these women dramatically reduces their chance of getting both ovarian and breast cancer. If women with gene mutations have had a breast cancer, oophorectomy reduces the chance of the cancer returning.

Suppression of the ovaries
LHRH agonists
Drugs have been developed that stop production of
the hormones that stimulate the ovaries to produce
oestrogen. These drugs are given by monthly injection
and their medical name is luteinising hormone-
releasing hormone agonists.

They can be used for women with early breast
cancer, as treatment after surgery or for women with
advanced breast cancer. The effects of these changes
are usually reversible when the drug is stopped.

Many women find that their periods do not return
immediately when they stop these drugs and it can
take many months or even years for periods to return.
The chance of you getting your periods back depends
on your age and what other treatment you have had.

These drugs are currently being investigated in
women with ER-negative cancers (tumours that are not
sensitive to oestrogen) who are having chemotherapy
to try to protect the ovaries from the effects of
chemotherapy. The hope is that, by switching off the
ovaries, there will be less damage by the
chemotherapy and this may allow women to maintain
their fertility even after chemotherapy.

The most common drug and the only one licensed
for breast cancer is goserelin (Zoladex). There are other
drugs available including buserelin (Prostap). The other
drugs are used mainly in prostate cancer but, as they
have an identical action to goserelin, doctors
occasionally prescribe them for breast cancer.

Goserelin is given as a monthly injection into the
lower abdomen, into the fat under skin below the
umbilicus (belly button). There is a three-monthly
injection available but it is not always effective in

women with breast cancer for the whole three-month period and is used mainly in men with prostate cancer.

LHRH agonists, when used in early breast cancer, are usually given for between two and five years to premenopausal women and can be given as an alternative to chemotherapy or after chemotherapy. They are often combined with other drugs such as tamoxifen or an aromatase inhibitor.

Drugs that interfere with the actions of hormones

Antioestrogens

Rather than stopping the production of oestrogen these drugs stop oestrogen getting to the oestrogen receptors where it works. These are often called antioestrogens.

The most common of these drugs is tamoxifen. Fulvestrant is another antioestrogen, which is occasionally used. Tamoxifen is a drug that has been widely used and has proved to be enormously successful for the treatment of women with ER-positive breast cancer in all ages and at all stages. The tamoxifen is taken as a once-daily tablet.

Tamoxifen

Tamoxifen given for five years to women with early breast cancer has been shown to reduce significantly the risk of recurrence and deaths from breast cancer, as well as the risk of developing a new cancer in the opposite breast.

Not all women who take tamoxifen benefit from it and one possible reason is that there is variation in how individuals handle tamoxifen when it gets into the body. Tamoxifen is converted after it has been absorbed to a more active antioestrogen. Some individuals convert more of the tamoxifen to the active form than others. Tests are being developed – those who are low converters get less benefit because they don't produce enough of the active form of tamoxifen for it to be effective. Low converters could then be given alternative drugs.

Tamoxifen is equally effective in pre- and postmenopausal women and in the latter it can be sequenced with the new aromatase inhibitors. Schedules include two years of tamoxifen followed by three years of an aromatase inhibitor or five years of tamoxifen followed by five years of an aromatase inhibitor.

Although tamoxifen has antioestrogen effects in the breast, in many other parts of the body its actions are similar to those of oestrogen. This has some benefits in that it preserves bone strength in postmenopausal women and lowers cholesterol, possibly reducing the risks of heart attack.

Side effects of tamoxifen
As it acts like oestrogen, it has some of the problems and complications that are seen in women who take hormone replacement therapy (HRT). The side effects of tamoxifen include:

- hot flushes

- vaginal discharge or irritation

- weight gain: randomised studies have not shown that women on tamoxifen gain more weight but weight gain is commonly reported by breast cancer patients on this drug

- increased joint pains

- eye problems: tamoxifen can slightly increase the risk of cataracts and another condition called iritis

- increased risk of deep venous thrombosis and pulmonary embolus (blood clots in the leg that can travel to the lungs); this is rare and the risk is thought only to be in postmenopausal women

- increased risk of developing endometrial cancer (cancer of the womb) in postmenopausal women; this type of cancer is rare but tamoxifen increases the likelihood that a woman will get endometrial cancer by about two to three times. For this reason any woman who develops vaginal bleeding on tamoxifen should be investigated.

Women should avoid becoming pregnant while they are taking tamoxifen because the effects on the baby are unknown. Women should use barrier forms of contraception because tamoxifen is a drug that has been shown to increase the likelihood of women getting pregnant – similar drugs to tamoxifen are used to treat infertility.

Fulvestrant
Fulvestrant is given as an injection into the buttock once a month. Studies are trying to find the best dose to use and are currently investigating higher doses – two injections every two weeks for the first month and then two injections monthly rather than the current once-a-month one-injection schedule that is in common use.

Fulvestrant is considered a 'pure' antioestrogen and does not have the same side effects as tamoxifen on the endometrium (lining of the womb) and does not seem to increase the risk of blood clots.

Aromatase inhibitors

These drugs interfere with the conversion of male hormones to female hormones. They are effective only in postmenopausal women and should not be used in premenopausal women. By reducing oestrogen production to extremely low levels, aromatase inhibitors deprive cancer cells of oestrogen, which results in the cancer cells dying and the cancer shrinking.

The aromatase inhibitors in common use are extremely specific and very effective and include anastrozole, letrozole and exemestane:

- Anastrozole in a dose of one milligram a day taken orally has been investigated extensively in both adjuvant treatment (treatment given in addition to primary therapy) to postmenopausal women and treatment of metastatic breast cancer (cancer that has spread). It appears to be somewhat more effective than tamoxifen.

- Letrozole given orally in a dose of two and a half milligrams per day has been shown to be considerably more effective than tamoxifen in metastatic breast cancer. Studies in early breast cancer have also suggested that it is more effective than tamoxifen when used as adjuvant therapy. Letrozole is widely used in women with large ER-positive breast cancers to shrink the cancer before surgery or to make a cancer that is not initially suitable for surgery operable. Studies have also shown that after five years of tamoxifen women who then take letrozole do better than those women who have no further treatment.

- Exemestane is the least commonly used of the aromatase inhibitors but is a very effective drug. The dose is 25 milligrams per day given orally. It can work in cancers that are resistant to letrozole or anastrozole. One study showed that women who took tamoxifen for two to three years and then switched to exemestane did much better than those women who continue on tamoxifen for five years.

Side effects of aromatase inhibitors
These drugs are generally well tolerated. It is likely that they all have slightly different side effects and, because a woman has side effects with one drug, it does not mean that she will get the same side effect with another aromatase inhibitor.

Hot flushes
Studies have tended to show that there are slightly fewer hot flushes with aromatase inhibitors than there are on tamoxifen.

Vaginal dryness
As there is no oestrogen present this can cause vaginal problems. Although dryness can be treated by local creams including oestrogen creams, the amount of oestrogen in these creams needs to be extremely low because studies have shown that some oestrogen preparations given vaginally can result in significant levels of oestrogen in the bloodstream.

Muscle and joint pains
These appear to be much more common with the aromatase inhibitors than with tamoxifen.

Fatigue
Some women do complain of feeling tired on these drugs.

Increased rates of fractures
As these drugs stop oestrogen production and oestrogen is important for bones, women who take these drugs have a slightly increased risk of bone fracture. Women who are taking these drugs for a long time should have their bone density checked and, if the bones are thin (osteoporotic), treatment with a bisphosphonate (bone-strengthening drug) is usually effective at strengthening the bones. Bisphosphonates can be taken with the aromatase inhibitors, so it is not necessary to stop this treatment even if osteoporosis develops.

Treating hot flushes in women on tamoxifen or aromatase inhibitors
Hot flushes tend to improve with time but can be extremely troublesome, particularly if they occur at night in association with night sweats. Wearing cool cotton clothing can help.

Megestrol acetate is a drug that acts in the body like the natural female hormone progesterone and can be effective in hot flushes. It is used at a low dose (20 mg daily) and is effective in controlling hot flushes in about 80 per cent of women.

There is no evidence that megestrol acetate increases the risk of recurrence of breast cancer and it certainly improves quality of life for women with hot flushes.

Drugs used to treat depression, including venlafaxine and fluoxetine, have been shown to be somewhat effective in hot flushes but fluoxetine may act by making tamoxifen less effective so caution is required.

A drug called gabapentin has been shown recently to improve hot flushes.

Although some women take soy (containing phyto-oestrogens) and believe that this improves hot flushes, there is concern that some soy products contain substantial amounts of oestrogen-like substances so these products are not therefore generally recommended for treating hot flushes in women with breast cancer.

Studies have shown no consistent benefit from vitamin E and evening primrose oil.

Clonidine is very occasionally effective but is not a very pleasant drug to take and it is rarely worth trying.

Studies of giving HRT to women have shown that it increases the risks of the cancer coming back, so it is not advised to give HRT to women with hormone-sensitive breast cancer.

Tibolone (Livial) is a drug that has oestrogen-like effects but is not actually an oestrogen. It does reduce hot flushes associated with tamoxifen but similar to HRT it increases the risk of cancer returning and so its use is not advised in women with breast cancer taking tamoxifen.

Choosing which hormone treatment to use
Premenopausal women

In premenopausal women the main options are an LHRH agonist plus tamoxifen or tamoxifen alone.

Hormone treatments

Hormonal treatment	Suitable for	How done/given
Removal of ovaries	Premenopausal women only	Surgery or radiotherapy
LHRH agonists	Premenopausal women only	Monthly injection in abdomen
Tamoxifen	Pre- and postmenopausal women	Daily tablet 20 mg
Fulvestrant	Postmenopausal women only	Monthly injection in one or both buttock
Aromatase inhibitors	Postmenopausal women if given alone Can be combined with LHRH agonist in premenopausal women	Daily tablet of anastrozole 1 mg, letrozole 2.5 mg, exemestane 25 mg

reatment length	Side effects
ermanent	Induction of menopause Vaginal dryness Hot flushes Osteoporosis
–5 years	As for removal of ovaries Pain and bruising at site of injection
Usually 5 years ometimes given for years followed by years of an romatase inhibitor n postmenopausal women	Venous thromboembolism Hot flushes Altered libido Gastrointestinal upset Vaginal discharge or dryness Menstrual disturbance Endometrial cancer Weight gain
Can be continued or as long as it is effective	Pain at the site of injection otherwise same as tamoxifen except does not cause venous thromboembolism or endometrial cancer
Usually 5 years unless used after 2 years amoxifen when 3 years used	Hot flushes (less than tamoxifen) Joint and muscle pains Osteoporosis Fatigue Vaginal dryness

Most women take tamoxifen and a few younger premenopausal women who still have regular periods will be advised to take tamoxifen combined with LHRH agonist.

Studies in younger women have investigated whether combining an LHRH agonist with an aromatase inhibitor is better than combining it with tamoxifen. It looks as though combining LHRH agonists with tamoxifen or the aromatase inhibitor anastrozole is equally effective.

Postmenopausal women
In postmenopausal women the choices are tamoxifen or the aromatase inhibitors. The current options are:

- five years of tamoxifen

- five years of an aromatase inhibitor

- two to three years of tamoxifen followed by two to three years of an aromatase inhibitor

- five years of tamoxifen followed by three years of an aromatase inhibitor

- two years of an aromatase inhibitor followed by three years of tamoxifen.

Deciding which treatment you should have depends on your general health and the risk of the cancer returning. If you have had a deep venous thrombosis or pulmonary embolus in the past, tamoxifen is not suitable and you will receive an aromatase inhibitor. Most women will now receive an aromatase inhibitor either immediately after surgery or after two to five years of tamoxifen.

Increasingly patients who have taken tamoxifen for two to three years are being switched to an aromatase inhibitor because studies have shown that this reduces cancer recurrence.

Nowadays most women who finish five years of tamoxifen will be advised to take an extra five years of treatment with letrozole because this not only reduces the chances of recurrence but also improves survival of women whose nodes were initially involved by cancer.

Chemotherapy after surgery (adjuvant chemotherapy)

Chemotherapy drugs are poisons that kill rapidly growing cells. Adjuvant chemotherapy is given to destroy any cancer cells that have escaped from the breast or the lymph glands to other parts of the body.

Even if all scans show that there is no evidence of any spread, it is known that in some women there are small groups of cancer cells that are undetectable and if these cancer cells are left untreated they can eventually cause problems. Chemotherapy can be given before or after surgery. When it is given after surgery, it is usually given immediately after surgery and before radiotherapy.

Chemotherapy and hormone therapy are not usually given together because chemotherapy is active against dividing or growing cells and hormone therapy switches off the growth of cells.

If you are to have chemotherapy and hormone therapy then the hormone therapy treatment will start after you have completed your chemotherapy.

Will I have chemotherapy?

The decision as to whether you have chemotherapy is based on:

- the size of the tumour

- whether the lymph nodes are involved

- the grade of the tumour

- the hormone receptor status of the tumour (ER positive or ER negative).

- whether the cancer is HER2 positive or negative (see page 212)

- your age and fitness.

Generally you are more likely to receive chemotherapy if:

- your tumour is large (over two centimetres)

- your lymph nodes are involved

- the tumour is grade 3 (see page 212)

- if the cancer is HER2 positive (see page 212)

- you are aged under 50 years

- the tumour is ER negative (see page 138).

If you have one or more of these features it is likely that you will be a good candidate for chemotherapy. Although chemotherapy is slightly more effective in ER-negative cancers, it is also effective in ER-positive cancers and further reduces the chances of the cancer coming back above and beyond that achieved with hormone therapy alone.

Intravenous chemotherapy

Sometimes chemotherapy is given before surgery, either to slow the growth of tumours that are growing rapidly or to shrink larger tumours. Chemotherapy, when given after surgery, usually starts before radiotherapy. Chemotherapy usually starts between three and four weeks after surgery, giving your body some time to recover from the effects of the operation.

Chemotherapy is most often given into a vein in your arm as a session of treatment, usually over a few hours. This is followed by a rest period usually of a few weeks, which allows your body to recover from any side effects of the treatment.

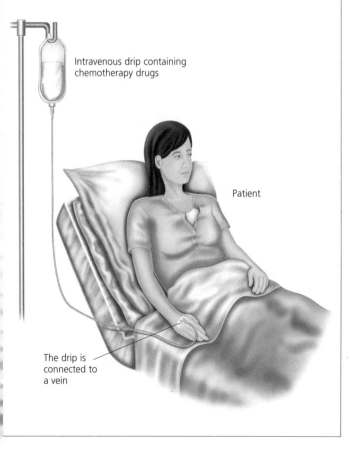

Intravenous drip containing chemotherapy drugs

Patient

The drip is connected to a vein

Benefits of chemotherapy

The benefit from chemotherapy depends partly on the risk of the cancer returning. Higher-risk women are more likely to get a benefit than lower-risk women.

Part of the effectiveness of chemotherapy in younger women is that it brings forward the age of menopause and so the ovaries stop producing oestrogen at a younger age than if no chemotherapy had been used.

Although chemotherapy appears to be effective in women of all ages its greatest benefit appears to be in younger women.

How is chemotherapy given?

Most women who receive chemotherapy will receive a combination of drugs. These are given as intravenous injections three weeks apart (a cycle). A course commonly consists of four, six, eight or even twelve cycles.

Commonly used drugs include anthracyclines, which have been shown to be one of the most effective types of drug in breast cancer; the most commonly used anthracyclines are doxorubicin (Adriamycin – A) and epirubicin (E). The anthracyclines are often combined with cyclophosphamide (C) and 5-fluorouracil (F) as CAF or FEC (the initials of the drugs). Other drugs in common use are the combination of cyclophosphamide, methotrexate and 5-fluorouracil, known as CMF.

Recently chemotherapy drugs called taxanes have been introduced in cancer treatment. They are derived from the bark of yew trees and there are two common agents in use: paclitaxel (Taxol) and docetaxel (Taxotere).

These drugs are used in women with metastatic breast cancer, but they are also used in some women with early breast cancer. The results from large studies of these drugs show a benefit in high-risk women so they are becoming increasingly used as part of adjuvant chemotherapy regimens.

Capecitabine is an oral drug that works similarly to 5-fluorouracil and is generally well tolerated; it has the obvious advantage of being in tablet form. Capecitabine is being tested after surgery and can be used either alone or in combination with other drugs in patients whose cancer has spread.

Commonly used regimens include the following:

- FEC: 5-fluorouracil, epirubicin and cyclophosphamide for six cycles

- CAF: cyclophosphamide, Adriamycin (doxorubicin) and 5-fluorouracil for four or six cycles

- Epi-CMF: three or four cycles of epirubicin or epirubicin followed by three or four cycles of CMF

- ACT: four cycles of doxorubicin (Adriamycin) and cyclophosphamide followed by three or four cycles of a taxane

- TAC: a taxane combined with doxorubicin (Adriamycin) and cyclophosphamide for six cycles

- AC: four cycles of Adriamycin (doxorubicin) and cyclophosphamide.

Other combinations are also used.

Chemotherapy before surgery (neoadjuvant chemotherapy)

Chemotherapy can also be given as initial treatment for larger or locally advanced breast cancers to shrink them down before surgery. This is known as neoadjuvant chemotherapy.

The advantages of neoadjuvant chemotherapy are that:

- a large tumour that would require a mastectomy to remove it may shrink sufficiently to allow lumpectomy or breast-conserving surgery

- if the cancer is locally advanced and not suitable for operation, the chemotherapy can make it operable

- if the tumour does respond and there is no cancer left after chemotherapy, this indicates that the long-term outlook is likely to be good

- if the drugs used are not effective, treatment can be changed.

Side effects of chemotherapy

Chemotherapy drugs are active against all dividing cells so tissues such as bone marrow, hair follicles, and the lining of the gut and bladder are all affected by chemotherapy and this explains why it causes unpleasant side effects. There are now treatments to combat most of these side effects.

Bone marrow suppression
Most chemotherapy drugs reduce the production of blood cells in the bone marrow. There are different types of cells in the blood and these include:

- white cells, which help fight off infection

- red cells, which carry oxygen round the body

- platelets, which are important for blood clotting.

If the production of any of these is markedly reduced by the chemotherapy, this could result in the problems listed below. If you develop any of these problems you should contact your doctor and get some advice.

A lowered resistance to infection

You will have blood counts taken before every cycle of chemotherapy. If your white count is low the chemotherapy may be put off, the dose may be reduced or you may be given a drug to stimulate white cell production.

The lowest levels of white count occur about seven to ten days after a dose of chemotherapy. It is very important if you feel hot or unwell and have any flu-like symptoms, including signs of fever, to contact the hospital immediately because these are signs of an infection.

If this happens, you usually have to go into hospital and receive antibiotics. If this happens for subsequent courses of chemotherapy a drug to stimulate your bone marrow to produce white cells can be given or the dose of the drug can be lowered to stop this happening again.

Anaemia (deficiency of red blood cells)

You can feel tired, lethargic, and dizzy and breathless if you are anaemic. If you are very anaemic this can be treated by a blood transfusion. Another option is to give you a drug called erythropoietin, which stimulates your bone marrow to produce more red cells.

Bruising/bleeding

Signs of a low platelet count include nosebleeds, bruising and unexplained bleeding. This can occur between cycles of chemotherapy and is a consequence of the effect of the chemotherapy on the production of platelets which play an important role in blood clotting.

Nausea and vomiting

These are very upsetting side effects and the doctors and nurses who give chemotherapy will work very hard at trying to prevent them. Anti-sickness medication will be started before you get chemotherapy and will continue for a few days afterwards. Even if you are feeling well you should take the medication because prevention is better than cure.

Sore mouth and mouth ulcers

This is a common complication of chemotherapy particularly after anthracyclines. It is important that you take great care about oral hygiene. Brush with a soft toothbrush and use mouthwashes after meals. Some people also complain of a dry mouth. You should avoid any major dental work while you are having chemotherapy.

Hair loss

This is almost inevitable with certain drugs including the anthracyclines and the taxanes. Scalp cooling can help reduce this but to be effective needs to be applied some time before chemotherapy is started and kept on for some time after it finishes.

There are two methods available to cool the scalp: one is to wear a 'cold cap' which is a cap containing gel that is cooled in the deep freeze; the second method blows very cold air on to your scalp.

Hair loss usually starts about two to three weeks after the first cycle of chemotherapy and by the second cycle most women will have lost all their hair.

Eyelashes, eyebrows and other body hair are also often affected. You should be fitted for a wig before chemotherapy begins.

Most women cope well with hair loss and find that it is not as bad as they thought it was going to be. Once your chemotherapy stops your hair will grow again but, when it comes in, it may be permanently softer and curly.

Premature menopause

Chemotherapy damages growing tissue including the ovaries and women who have chemotherapy are likely to have the menopause at a younger age. Even if your periods do not start after you have completed chemotherapy, it does not mean that you are postmenopausal.

In some women there is a gap of many months after the end of chemotherapy before menstruation returns. Chemotherapy will reduce the chances of you being able to become pregnant in the future.

If you are thinking of having children it is important to discuss this with your doctor before you start chemotherapy. There are ways of storing eggs or part of the ovary to try to get round this problem. Ongoing studies are looking at whether LHRH analogues can protect the ovaries from the effects of chemotherapy.

Although most women stop their periods during chemotherapy, it is important to realise that there is a small chance of you becoming pregnant while on chemotherapy, so you need to ensure that you take precautions and use barrier methods of contraception.

Fatigue

All chemotherapy causes women to be fatigued and tired. This is the side effect that women complain of most. It is important to realise that during chemotherapy you will not be able to do the things that you could before.

It does not mean, however, that you should stop going out. You may need to cut down on the amount that you would normally do but you should take regular exercise. Because you tend to do less this may cause weight gain so regular exercise (swimming or walking) will help to limit the weight that you might gain during treatment and will also improve your energy levels. The problem with fatigue is that it often continues even after you have finished your chemotherapy and in some women it can last for many years.

Diarrhoea

Some women develop this but it can usually be controlled by medication.

Constipation

This is the most common side effect of the drugs given to stop sickness. It is important that you keep drinking and eat a well-balanced diet when you are having chemotherapy because this is the best way to stop this problem.

Thrombosis and pulmonary embolus

Women who have chemotherapy are at slightly increased risk of these complications. If you have any leg swelling or any breathlessness you should report this to your doctor immediately.

Problems with veins

Chemotherapy is given through the veins in the back of the hand. If you have had removal of all the axillary nodes from one side, chemotherapy is usually given into the opposite hand.

Once you inject chemotherapy into a vein, it damages the vein. This can result in the vein becoming sore and/or hardened and the blood stops flowing in the vein. This settles down over a few weeks.

Chemotherapy is usually given via a drip and it is important to ensure that the chemotherapy does not leak out from the vein into the tissues. Chemotherapy is given by experienced nurses and doctors who are aware of this problem.

Damage to your heart

Doxorubicin (Adriamycin) and to a lesser extent epirubicin can damage the heart if given in high doses. Doctors are aware of this and calculate carefully the dose so that you are unlikely to develop this problem. Sometimes before chemotherapy a heart scan is performed to check how effectively your heart is pumping.

A particular problem has been found in women given a combination of anthracyclines and the drug trastuzumab (Herceptin – see below). If you are getting this combination you will have a heart scan before treatment and you will also have regular scans during treatment to make sure that no damage develops.

Cystitis
Some drugs, especially cyclophosphamide, can cause irritation of the bladder (cystitis). This is usually prevented by drinking regular fluids.

Damage to nerves
The taxanes can cause damage to nerves of the hands and feet and this can cause pain, tingling or numbness. Report this to your doctor if this develops.

Redness of the hands and feet
5-Fluorouracil given intravenously and oral capecitabine (Xelda) can cause the palms of the hands and the soles of the feet to become red and sore.

Skin and nail changes
You may develop dry and flaky skin on your hands and feet after several cycles. Your skin will also be more sensitive to sunlight with a tendency to sunburn. Your nails can become discoloured.

Red urine
Epirubicin is red and you may notice that your urine is red for up to 24 hours after each injection

Dizziness/hot flush
These can sometimes occur when cyclophosphamide is injected.

Temporary taste changes
These can occur throughout treatment. Sharp and spicy foods often taste better than bland foods! Some patients lose their sense of taste.

Trastuzumab

Trastuzumab (Herceptin) is a newer type of drug that is given to women whose cancers have a lot of receptors for HER2 on the surface of their cancer cells. These cancers are known as HER2 positive. HER2 is a growth factor that combines with other members of the HER family (HER1, -3 or -4) to cause cancer cells to grow (see page 81).

Trastuzumab is a particular type of drug known as a monoclonal antibody and the antibody binds to the HER2 on the surface of the cancer cell and stops it combining with other members of the HER group, which it does to keep the cancer cells active. Trastuzumab stops the cell growing and then the cancer cells eventually die.

Women who have cancers that are HER2 positive tend to have faster-growing cancers. Giving trastuzumab after surgery together with chemotherapy for early breast cancer significantly reduces the chances of the cancer returning (by up to 50 per cent).

Trastuzumab can also be given before surgery combined with chemotherapy and is very effective in shrinking down large HER2-positive breast cancers before surgery.

It is an expensive treatment. It is licensed to be given only at the same time as or after chemotherapy. Trastuzumab is given after surgery for one year. For women whose cancer has spread but is controlled by trastuzumab the drug is continued while the cancer is under control, which in some women is for more than five years. Trastuzumab can be given at the same time or after chemotherapy.

Side effects

Trastuzumab can affect the heart particularly when combined with anthracycline chemotherapy (see page 152). For this reason you will have a heart scan before and during treatment. If the scan shows that the function of the heart has been affected, you may need to discontinue the drug for a period. The heart function usually picks up again to allow completion of the whole course, which consists of 17 injections 3 weeks apart.

Occasionally patients have an allergic reaction to trastuzumab. If this happens it does so shortly after starting the injection and is very treatable. After the first few injections you can usually have the rest of the course at home. There are very few other side effects. It is a new generation of targeted therapies and is very safe and very effective.

Lapatanib

This is a new drug that can be taken in tablet form, and is also effective against HER2-positive cancers. It can be effective when trastuzumab has stopped working. Studies are under way to find out how it can most effectively be incorporated into treatment plans.

Pertuzumab

This is another monoclonal antibody that targets HER1, HER2 and HER3, and is currently undergoing clinical trials.

Bisphosphonates

These are drugs that inhibit bone resorption and are used in the treatment of osteoporosis. Early trials suggested that women with breast cancer who took bisphosphonates after surgery had a small but significant improvement in survival. More recent trials with a new more potent drug, zoledronate, which is given by a 15-minute infusion every few months, have confirmed the benefit of these drugs in improving survival. Further studies have been performed and the results of these are awaited.

If they confirm the benefit, then it is likely that these drugs will become part of the routine treatment after surgery for certain groups of women. The length of time that the treatment needs to continue is still being assessed. Bisphosphonates reduce the bone loss associated with the use of the aromatase inhibitors. Patients taking an aromatase inhibitor should be considered for a dual energy X-ray absorptiometry (DEXA) scan to check bone density. Those with osteoporosis at diagnosis or who have major bone loss during treatment should be considered for bisphosphonate therapy. Oral bisphosphonates are available but are not always easy to take and can cause heartburn. A major potential side effect is damage to the jawbone but this is very rare and occurs only in patients who have dental problems, where the bone has been damaged or is left uncovered after dental surgery or infection.

Immunotherapy

Stimulating the body to kill the cancer through activating the body's immune system has been a goal of treatment for many years. Drugs are in trials and vaccines against cancers are being developed. As yet, none of the attempts to stimulate the immune system has proved very effective.

PARP inhibitors

When a cell divides and forms two cells, the genetic material in the cell has to be copied. The body has three mechanisms to check that the cells produced are perfect copies. In *BRCA*-1 and *BRCA*-2 gene carriers, a faulty gene for one of three mechanisms is inherited from either the mother or the father. In each cell there are two copies of each gene. If the normal copy of the *BRCA*-1 or *BRCA*-2 gene becomes faulty, then the gene does not function.

Thus if your *BRCA*-1 or *BRCA*-2 genes are faulty, you are much more likely to produce a faulty copy each time that a breast cell divides. Some but not all the faults that are not detected because of loss of *BRCA*-1 or *BRCA*-2 result in the development of a breast cancer. When they divide, cancer cells are much more likely to copy abnormally and produce faulty copies, but these are usually picked up and repaired.

In a woman or man with a cancer who is a *BRCA*-1 or *BRCA*-2 carrier, the knocking out of one of the other mechanisms for checking that cell copies are perfect results in the cancer cells having only one of the three checking mechanisms. As the cancer cells divide abnormally and the faults are no longer repaired, the cancer cells produced have so many faults that they die. The drugs that knock out one of the other checking mechanisms are called PARP inhibitors. They are currently undergoing clinical trials but show great promise in patients with cancer who are *BRCA*-1 or *BRCA*-2 carriers, and also in triple-negative breast cancer.

Other new drugs

There are lots of other drugs being studied in clinical trials (see next chapter).

KEY POINTS

■ Drugs used to treat breast cancer include hormone treatments, chemotherapy and new biologic therapies

■ Hormone treatments act on the main female hormone oestrogen which in most breast cancers stimulates them to grow

■ The most commonly used hormone treatment has been tamoxifen and this is usually given for about five years

■ Aromatase inhibitors are used alone or together in sequence with tamoxifen in postmenopausal women with hormone receptor-positive breast cancers

■ Side effects of hormone treatment include menopausal symptoms, tiredness and joint pains

■ Chemotherapy kills rapidly growing cells

■ Treatments are usually given by injection with six to eight doses or cycles being given every three weeks

■ Side effects of chemotherapy include reduced resistance to infection, sickness, hair loss and tiredness

■ Trastuzumab is effective in the 15 to 20 per cent of women whose cancers are HER2 positive

New developments and clinical trials

Can a cure be found?

In most major breast units, research into finding better ways of treating breast cancer is going on all the time. As none of the current treatments results in a cure for all patients, doctors in these units are looking continually for new and better ways to treat breast cancer.

Clinical trials

One way of investigating treatments is through clinical trials that involve trying out new drugs in patients. Before a clinical trial takes place on a drug a lot of early work and tests are performed.

If the early work suggests that the new treatment might be better than the current standard treatment, doctors carry out trials to compare the new treatment with the best available standard treatment. This is called a controlled clinical trial and is the only reliable way of testing a new treatment.

Usually these trials are carried out in several hospitals around the country to get enough patients into the trial. To make sure that the results are not biased, often you and your doctor will not know whether you are taking the new drug or the standard treatment.

Taking part in a clinical trial

In randomised controlled clinical trials some patients will receive the best standard treatment and others will receive the new treatment.

In such a trial you cannot choose which treatment you receive; a computer assigns you to the standard or the new treatment. This method of randomisation ensures that equal numbers of patients get both treatments and removes bias.

Eventually, when the trial is completed it is possible to tell whether the new treatment is any better than the standard treatment.

It is important to realise that not all trials show that the new treatment is better. If you enter a trial and do not get the new treatment, you should not be too disappointed. If you do not receive the test treatment in the trial you will receive the best standard treatment, which is what you would have had if you had not entered the trial.

Before any trials are allowed to take place, the trial needs to be approved by an ethics committee. Patients also need to sign an informed consent form before entering any clinical trial. This consent means that patients know what the trial is about, understand why it is being conducted and why they have been invited to take part.

Clinical trials

Phase 1
A small number of healthy volunteers, usually between 10 and 12 people, are selected for the first set of trials. These tests work out whether the medicine is safe.

Phase 2
Trials are designed to see if a new medicine works in a small number of patients with the condition or disease being tested. Between 100 and 200 patients are selected and monitored to see if they have mild or severe side effects.

Phase 3
The largest number of patients so far is selected (perhaps between 1,000 and 3,000) to take the medicine under medical supervision for approximately six months. Phase 3 trials are usually carried out in a hospital or clinic setting and may involve a number of different countries.

If the results are satisfactory, they will be presented to the licensing and other relevant authorities who decide whether or not to give them a licence.

Phase 4
Even when newly licensed medicines are launched, they are still tested and many thousands of patients help to continue the research and help doctors. Doctors are looking to see how the new medicine is used in a real-life situation, when a patient is at home or work. If the medicine has a very rare side effect, for example a reaction that will affect one person in 50,000 taking the medicine, then it is extremely unlikely that these side effects will be discovered until after the new medicine is available to be prescribed.

Even after patients agree to take part in the trial they can withdraw at any stage if they change their mind. Importantly your decision as to whether to enter or withdraw from the trial will not affect your treatment or your doctor's attitude towards you.

KEY POINTS

- Trials of new drugs are going on all the time to try to improve the outcome of treatment for breast cancer

- If you are asked to take part in such a trial your decision will not affect your treatment or your doctor's attitude to you

- If you enter a trial you can withdraw at any time without giving a reason

What happens if breast cancer returns?

Types of recurrence

There are different ways of classifying recurrent cancers; the one that is in most common use splits cancers into:

1 Local recurrence in the area around the breast and the axilla

2 Recurrence elsewhere in the body, which is known as a secondary growth or metastasis.

Local recurrence

If you develop local recurrence and have no disease elsewhere in the body, it is usually possible just to remove this by surgery. If surgery is performed it will often be combined with radiotherapy and/or, if you have not had it previously, a change in drug treatment if you are taking hormonal drugs. Radiotherapy without surgery is used in some women who have not had this treatment to the area before.

Chemotherapy or newer biologic treatments may be used and can be given before or after surgery and/or radiotherapy.

The first sign of local recurrence is usually a lump in the breast, or in the skin of the breast, the armpit or in or close to the scar where you had your surgery. It is important if you do develop a lump or nodule in your breast at or around your scar or armpit to get this checked by your doctor.

Metastatic breast cancer

In some women cancer cells break away from the primary breast cancer and spread to other parts of the body forming so-called metastases.

These cells survive because they are resistant to the adjuvant hormone therapy and chemotherapy and so survive despite these therapies. They can lie dormant for many years and even decades before they start to grow.

In a few women there will be signs that the cancer has spread at the time they are first diagnosed. This will be evident because of abnormalities on X-rays or scans. The common sites for breast cancer to spread to are bone, liver, lungs and brain.

The treatments available include:

- hormonal therapy

- chemotherapy

- radiotherapy

- monoclonal antibody therapy – trastuzumab (Herceptin).

The best treatment for you will depend on:

- which parts of the body are affected by breast cancer

- whether you have had your menopause

- the treatment that you have had in the past

- your age and general health

- whether the cancer cells are hormone receptor positive

- whether the cancer cells are HER2 positive.

The treatment that you will receive is the one that is most likely to control the breast cancer and cause the fewest side effects. With cancer that has spread the aim of treatment is to control the cancer for as long as possible, improve any symptoms and prolong length of life. Most treatments are effective at shrinking the cancer or stopping its growth. Although cure is not expected, control of the disease is usually possible.

The same drug treatments used for early breast cancer are also used for cancer that has spread. This includes hormonal therapies, chemotherapy and biologic therapies such as trastuzumab. In some women the cancer has spread to only one specific site, whereas, in others, tests show that the cancer involves multiple sites. There are specific treatments for cancers that have spread to involve specifically the bones, lungs and brain.

Treatment of metastases
Bone metastases
X-rays of the bones, a bone scan, a CT scan or MR scan are the tests used to diagnose bone metastases.

The bones are the most common site to which breast cancers spread. The most common symptom is pain. This pain can usually be controlled by a combination of painkillers and radiotherapy.

If the bone is particularly weak and likely to break or if the bone has already broken, surgery can be effective at strengthening, repairing or replacing the affected bone.

Another effective treatment for cancer that has spread to bones is to give a bisphosphonate. These are bone-strengthening agents and stop the cancer cells damaging bone. Bisphosphonates are usually given as an intravenous injection every few weeks. Newer drugs take about 15 minutes to give. They reduce pain in the bones and strengthen the bone so reducing the chances of getting a fracture.

One recognised complication of advanced breast cancer is the production of too much calcium from the bones, called hypercalcaemia. Symptoms of hyper-calcaemia include nausea (feeling sick), abdominal pain, constipation, fatigue, confusion and drowsiness.

The best treatment for this is to flush the calcium out of the body by setting up a drip and giving fluid into the veins combined with regular bisphosphonates.

Lung metastases
These are diagnosed by a chest X-ray or CT scan of the chest. There are two types of involvement of the lung by breast cancer.

Outer lining of the lung
The most common is disease affecting the outer lining of the lung, known as the pleura, which results in fluid collecting around the lung, causing breathlessness. This is known as a pleural effusion.

Simple drainage is effective at removing the fluid but after simple drainage the fluid tends to re-collect. Draining the fluid by placing a drain between the ribs into the fluid and leaving it in for two or three days is effective at draining off the fluid and in many patients stops the fluid coming back.

People who get recurrent build-up of fluid benefit from injection of talc or a chemotherapy agent called bleomycin into the space between the chest wall and lungs, where the fluid builds up. This causes the lungs to stick to the chest wall and can stop the fluid continuing to collect.

Within the lung

If the lung itself is affected the symptoms include breathlessness and/or a cough. Cough medicines are often effective at controlling this symptom. Breathlessness caused by disease in the lungs is best treated by switching treatment to another chemotherapy drug(s) or another hormone drug.

Brain metastases

These can be diagnosed on a CT or MR scan of the brain. Symptoms of spread to the brain include nausea, vomiting, fatigue, weakness, feeling unsteady on your feet, double vision and fits. Some women get headaches that are worse in the morning, but most women with breast cancer who develop headaches do not have cancer spread to the brain.

Initial treatment is with steroids, which reduces swelling in the brain and improves symptoms. This is usually followed by radiotherapy.

When cure is not possible

If it is not possible to stop the cancer completely, it is nearly always possible to control symptoms such as pain and nausea. Most hospitals have a specialised palliative care team who can advise your GP or the hospital oncology department about the optimal use of drugs to help you.

These will probably include painkillers and drugs that combat nausea and diarrhoea. They can also advise on how to improve your appetite, which can often be poor as a result of the illness or the treatment.

Coping with recurrent or metastatic breast cancer

Many women find it even more difficult to face cancer that returns (secondary breast cancer) than they did when they were first diagnosed. Having been well for so long it is difficult to face going through further treatment that can be unpleasant.

You will need the support of your friends and family through this difficult time. Support is also available from your surgeon, oncologist, breast care nurse, GP and many self-help groups.

Some patients get support from Macmillan and Marie Curie nurses who come out and visit at home. A variety of organisations and self-help groups that also provide support are listed in 'Further information' on page 220.

KEY POINTS

■ Breast cancer can return in the breast/chest area and armpit (local recurrence) or elsewhere in the body (metastatic or secondary breast cancer)

■ The most common sites of spread of breast cancer are bone, liver, lungs and brain

■ When cure is no longer possible a variety of treatments is available to keep patients pain free and to control any symptoms from the cancer

■ Similar treatments are used to those for treating early breast cancer but with metastatic cancer cure is not expected

■ There are specific treatments that are effective at controlling disease in the bone, lungs and brain

Reconstruction

Breast reconstruction
What is breast reconstruction?

Breast reconstruction is an operation to recreate the shape of a breast that has been removed by mastectomy (removal of the whole breast) or lumpectomy (removal of part of the breast).

The aim of reconstruction is to restore the shape of the breast and to match the opposite breast as closely as possible. There are different ways of doing this and the type of operation that you have will depend on:

- the type of disease that you have in your breast

- the operation you have had, whether a mastectomy or breast-conserving surgery (lumpectomy)

- whether radiotherapy has been given previously or is planned after this operation

- your health and general fitness

- your choice and preference.

As well as reconstructing the breast, it is also possible to reconstruct the nipple and the surrounding area, which is known as the areola.

It is important to realise that, even if you have a breast reconstruction that matches the other breast, it will never feel the same as the other breast. Also, any nipple that is reconstructed will not have the same sensation as your normal nipple.

Why women choose reconstruction

There are clearly some benefits from having reconstruction and there are also some risks. The following are the benefits:

- You will have increased freedom of dress. If you have a mastectomy and immediate breast reconstruction you may not have to worry about different bras or changing your wardrobe at all.

- You will not have to wear an external prosthesis.

- Women who have had a reconstruction say that generally they feel more confident and better about their bodies compared with women who do not have one.

Problems with reconstruction

Although your shape can be restored, it will not feel like a normal breast and a reconstructed breast often sits a little higher and is firmer than the opposite breast.

Breast reconstruction is not usually one operation. To get a good match between the two breasts, it is usually necessary for patients to have two or three operations. This can involve making the opposite breast smaller, lifting it or making it bigger. It may also be necessary at a second operation to tidy up scars on the reconstructed breast or to make minor adjustments to improve its shape.

There is absolutely no evidence that having a breast reconstruction increases the chance of cancer coming back and it does not make any recurrence of cancer more difficult to detect.

If you are interested in breast reconstruction you need to discuss this with your doctor. If you have been told that you need a mastectomy you should be offered the option of breast reconstruction as long as you are fit enough.

Your surgeon might indicate to you that if you want reconstruction this would be better carried out as a delayed procedure six to twelve months after the mastectomy rather than immediately.

The reasons for this may be because it is planned to give you radiotherapy after mastectomy or some of the skin of the breast that is affected or dimpled by the cancer needs to be removed by the surgeon and this might make reconstruction technically difficult.

Timing of breast reconstruction

Breast reconstruction in the UK is most commonly carried out at the time of initial surgery. If you are having a mastectomy, the whole breast can be reconstructed. If you are having a large part of the breast removed, part of the breast can be replaced using muscle or tissue from elsewhere in the body.

If you have had a mastectomy in the past you may be a candidate for reconstruction. This is called delayed reconstruction. Also, if you have had a lumpectomy. but your treated breast does not match your other breast because it is smaller or an abnormal shape, it is possible to perform a partial breast reconstruction and reshape the treated breast to match it to the opposite side.

If you are having immediate reconstruction at the time of mastectomy it can take longer to organise than a straightforward mastectomy. This should not put you off because delaying surgery by a week or two will not make any difference to your outcome.

If there is going to be a delay, check with your surgeon about whether you should start some drug treatment before the operation. If your cancer is hormone sensitive, taking tamoxifen in premenopausal women or a drug such as letrozole (see page 142) in postmenopausal women before surgery can help control the cancer and even shrink it.

Where can you have a reconstruction?

Most breast units offer immediate reconstruction. This surgery is performed either by a specialist breast surgeon who is trained in both cancer surgery and reconstructive surgery or by two surgeons, the operation to remove the cancer being performed by a breast surgeon and the reconstruction surgery by a plastic surgeon.

If you are having reconstruction it is important to ask your surgeon and breast care nurse to show you photographs of the probable results. You may also be able to get the name and telephone number of a patient who has had this procedure so that you can talk to her. You can get further information on reconstruction from some of the self-help groups such as Breast Cancer Care (see page 221).

What are the types of reconstruction?

There are three main ways in which the breast can be reconstructed:

1 Using an implant alone.

2 Swinging in tissue from your back or your abdomen (tummy). This tissue is left attached to its blood supply and is known as a pedicled flap. The muscle with overlying skin and fat from the back or the abdomen is used either alone or together with an implant to reconstruct the breast.

3 Tissue taken from the abdomen or the buttock region is detached from its blood supply and transferred and attached to a new blood supply in the armpit or under the ribcage to create a new breast. These procedures are known as free flaps and require microsurgery. They are usually performed only by specially trained plastic surgeons.

Breast implants

Breast implants have been used for many years. Most implants are a silicone shell filled with silicone although they can also be filled with saline (salt water).

Although saline implants sound attractive they do not have a natural feel and give a much less realistic reconstruction than silicone implants. Saline implants are also more likely to leak and wrinkle and interfere with the reading of mammograms. For that reason, most surgeons do not use saline implants.

Silicone implants are essentially bags of silicone gel enclosed in a thin silicone rubber outer shell. Silicone is used because it is soft and flexible and feels like natural breast tissue.

Early implants

Implants have changed over the years. Originally the implants that were first used had a thick outer shell and contained thick silicone. These did not feel breast like.

They were quickly replaced by second-generation implants, which contained more fluid silicone and had a very thin smooth-walled shell. The outer shell of these second-generation implants tended to wear out over 10 to 20 years and so with time these implants ruptured or leaked.

Most controversy and problems with breast implants have surrounded the use of these second-generation implants.

Modern implants

The silicone implants that are used now have a rough (textured) outer surface that stops them moving and they have a much thicker shell than the second-generation implants.

The silicone gel that is currently used is often solid silicone gel rather than liquid silicone gel. This means that, if the implant is cut in two, the two pieces remain intact and do not leak.

Silicone injections

The biggest problems reported with silicone are not related to silicone implants but because liquid silicone was injected into the breasts in some women. This was rarely carried out in the UK and silicone injections into the breast are now banned.

Safety of implants

Although there have been lots of reports that silicone

implants cause other health problems, all the research that has been performed has shown no link between these implants and the development of any disease.

Silicone implants were banned for several years in the USA but they are now in use again. In the UK the Department of Health has asked medical specialists on three occasions over recent years to look at the safety of silicone implants. The last report in July 1998 concluded that there was no good evidence that silicone implants cause any significant disease including arthritis.

How long do silicone implants last?
The average lifespan of a second-generation implant is about 15 years. By this time about half the implants are either leaking or ruptured.

The new implants that are now in use will almost certainly last much longer and it is currently believed that these implants will last between 20 and 25 years.

What happens if my implant leaks?
It is very rare that, if an implant leaks, any silicone leaks outside the capsule that the body forms around it. If an implant rupture is suspected because of a change in shape of the breast or because a mammogram indicates a possible leak this can be confirmed by ultrasound or magnetic resonance imaging (MRI). The body can react to silicone that has leaked from implants by forming lumps which can be painful.

If the MR scan shows that the implant has ruptured but there is no silicone leaking outside the capsule, it is usual to have the implant removed, the silicone washed out and the implant replaced, but it is not absolutely necessary. The operation to remove the implant usually removes the capsule around the implant to make sure that all the silicone is removed from the body.

Breast reconstruction using implants alone

When reconstruction using implants was first introduced it was common to use implants after a mastectomy to try to produce an immediate breast

Breast implants

Breast implants are made of an outer layer of silicone and an inner part which is filled either with saline (salt water) or silicone gel. Silicone and saline have so far been shown to be effective and safe. The outer layer is made of a material called silicone elastomer, a material similar to rubber to reduce the risk of leakage.

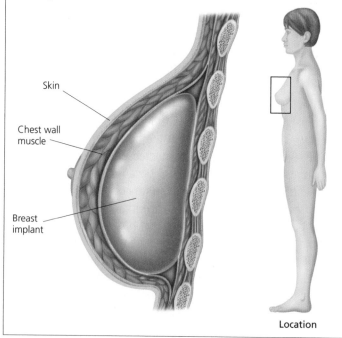

Skin

Chest wall muscle

Breast implant

Location

reconstruction. The implant was placed either under the skin or underneath the chest wall muscle next to the ribs.

Unfortunately reconstruction using implants alone is suitable only for women with small breasts and the final result from this type of reconstruction is not generally as good as that using skin and muscle from the back or abdomen.

The scar from this type of reconstruction usually runs from side to side or, if the nipple is left, it may run under the nipple.

Breast reconstruction using tissue expanders

Once some of the skin of the breast is removed, it is difficult to get the reconstructed breast to match the opposite breast, unless extra skin is produced by stretching the skin and muscle that is already there.

Breast reconstruction using a tissue expander places an expandable implant under the muscle of the chest wall; the expander is attached by a tube to an injection port that sits under the skin placed either below or at the side of the expander or the injection port is integrated into the expander.

This port is used to allow filling and stretching of the skin and chest wall muscle. To allow more rapid expansion of the muscle it is possible to sew in a layer of tissue which is an acellular dermal matrix derived from donated human or pig skin. This results in better expansion of the lower part of the breast where it is needed.

Fluid is injected into the implant over a few months. This results in the tissues stretching and new skin develops in the same way as a woman develops extra skin on her abdomen when she is pregnant. Fluid injection causes some discomfort but this usually settles very quickly.

Reconstruction using tissue expanders

After breast surgery, a patient may choose reconstructive surgery. One option involves inserting an implant under the skin and chest wall muscle. This is expanded over several months by injecting saline into it.

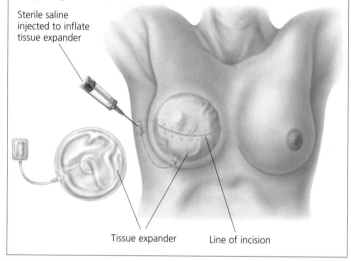

Sterile saline injected to inflate tissue expander

Tissue expander   Line of incision

The inflatable silicone bag is left in place for several months until the tissues have stretched to produce a good match to the opposite breast.

Then a second operation is performed to remove the tissue expander and replace it with a permanent implant.

Some tissue expanders have two spaces within the implant. The outer space is filled with silicone gel and the inner balloon is filled with saline. These devices are slightly over-inflated (blown up) to larger than the planned final volume over several weeks and then some of the salt water is removed through the valve to produce a breast reconstruction that matches the opposite natural breast as closely as possible.

Reconstruction using tissue matrix

1. An expandable implant is placed under the muscle of the chest wall. This is used to fill and stretch the skin and chest wall muscle.
To allow more rapid expansion of the muscle it is possible to sew in a layer of tissue derived from human or pig skin. Alloderm is human skin that is treated to remove the risk of rejection or inflammation. Permacol and Strattice are pig rather than human skin.

The benefit of Alloderm, Permacol or Strattice is to give support to the implant which may help prevent bottoming out (downward movement of the implant) or extrusion of the implant through the skin

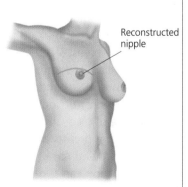

Muscles

Expandable implant

Alloderm

2. The inflatable silicone bag is left in place for several months until the tissues have stretched to produce a good match to the opposite breast. Then a second operation is performed to remove the tissue expander and replace it with a permanent implant

After expander exchange for implant

Reconstructed nipple

3. Final appearance with nipple

An advantage of these devices, which are called Becker expander prostheses, is that they do not need to be removed and can be left in permanently. All the surgeon needs to do is to remove the filler port and the tubing that connects the port to the implant.

Use of implants or tissue expanders is not usually suitable for people who have had radiotherapy. This is because radiotherapy damages the skin and does not allow the skin to stretch as easily. For women who have had radiotherapy, therefore, a reconstruction using skin, muscle and fat from elsewhere is usually required. With the use of tissue matrix (see page 185), it is sometimes possible to get a good quality reconstruction even after radiotherapy.

Breast reconstruction using muscle and skin flaps

This type of reconstruction uses muscle, skin and underlying fat from different parts of the body and transfers them to the breast to create a satisfactory breast shape. This type of surgery is known as flap surgery.

The tissue most commonly used is from either the back or the abdomen – areas of the body that contain large muscles and can provide enough skin, fat and muscle with a good blood supply to help create a reasonable breast shape. The large muscle from the back is called latissimus dorsi and the muscle from the abdomen is rectus abdominis.

Flap reconstructions are now the most commonly used type of reconstruction. These flaps can be used to create larger breasts and are particularly appropriate for women who have had radiotherapy. This type of reconstruction can take many hours to perform and usually requires a stay in hospital of five days or more.

Latissimus dorsi flap with an implant

There is a broad thick muscle that lies directly under the skin on each side of your back called latissimus dorsi. The muscle used to reconstruct a breast is taken from the same side of the body as the breast that has been removed (that is, a right-sided mastectomy would involve removal of the skin and muscle from the right side of the back).

There are other layers of muscle in the back and, although removal of a muscle can result in a slight weakness, in general other muscles compensate for the lost muscle so that you should not notice too much difference during everyday activities.

The skin and underlying fat remain attached to the muscle, which is kept attached to its own blood supply, and the flap is tunnelled through the armpit to create a new breast shape.

Usually the amount of skin that is removed from the back is more than the amount of skin removed at the time of mastectomy and some of the skin can be buried to produce a satisfactory size and shape, so it is generally possible to get a very good match with the opposite breast.

It is not always possible to get enough tissue from the back to fill the whole breast, so a small implant is often placed underneath the muscle to produce a reconstructed breast of the same volume as the opposite normal breast.

This type of operation leaves scars on the back and on the reconstructed breast. The scar on the back is usually positioned so that it will lie under the bra strap. Some surgeons prefer to leave a more diagonal scar. This can make it more difficult to cover up but these types of scars are usually covered by garments such as swimsuits.

Reconstruction using muscle and skin from the back

1. This operation involves moving a large muscle (latissimus dorsi) and some overlying fat and skin from the back of your body

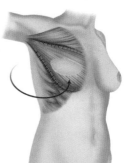

Preoperative surgical markings on section to transfer

Area of skin to be removed

Latissimus dorsi muscle

2. The flap and its blood supply are tunnelled under the skin just below the armpit. It is then put into position to make a new breast shape

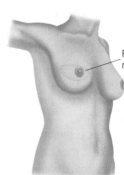

The flap is transferred in the operating theatre

3. Final appearance with nipple reconstruction

Reconstructed nipple

The reason for using a diagonal scar is that it can give more skin. The scar on the breast can be very small if the reconstruction is being performed at the same time as the mastectomy because skin can be spared at the mastectomy, but there will be more scarring if you have a delayed reconstruction, because more skin is required to create a satisfactory breast shape after a previous mastectomy.

Lower abdominal tissue
This uses the rectus abdominis muscle and skin and fat from the abdomen. This is known as a transverse rectus abdominis myocutaneous flap reconstruction, sometimes referred to as a TRAM because a **t**ransverse piece of skin is used and the **r**ectus **a**bdominis **m**uscle is used.

In this operation fat, usually with underlying muscle and overlying skin from the lower part of the abdomen, is used to reconstruct the breast.

The flap can be rotated and tunnelled upwards leaving it attached to the body; this is called a pedicled flap.

Alternatively, it can be removed completely from the body and reattached to a new blood supply in the breast region – a so-called free flap.

TRAM flaps are usually big enough in volume to match the opposite breast and an implant is rarely needed. The scar on the abdomen is usually horizontal and just below the bikini line. During the operation the umbilicus (belly button) is repositioned.

In a free flap the same skin and fat from the lower abdomen are used but less muscle is taken. The blood vessels supplying the flap are identified and then cleaned and cut and are later rejoined to blood vessels either under the arm or under the breastbone.

Reconstruction using a pedicled TRAM flap

This type of operation is referred to as a pedicled TRAM flap because the transverse rectus abdominis muscle is used. TRAM may be done as either a pedicle flap (which means the tissue is pulled under the skin and attached in the chest area without cutting its blood supply) or a free flap (which means that the tissue and blood vessels are cut and reattached in the chest area).

1. A flap of fat and some muscle with its blood vessels, together with overlying skin, is taken from the abdomen (tummy)

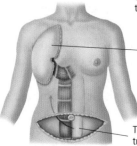

Transverse rectus abdominis muscle

Preoperative surgical markings on section to transfer

2. The flap is then tunnelled upwards from the abdomen and attached to the chest wall to create the shape of a breast

Flap is reattached at predetermined site

The flap is transferred in the operating threatre

3. Final appearance with nipple reconstruction. This method usually gives enough tissue to match the remaining breast, so an implant is not usually needed

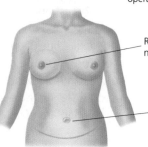

Reconstructed nipple

Navel (belly button) is repositioned and stitched at its new site

Reconstruction using a 'free' TRAM flap

Again the transverse rectus abdominis muscle is used but this time it is removed completely from the body and reattached to a new blood supply in the breast region – a so-called free flap.

1. A flap of fat and some muscle together with overlying skin are surgically removed from the abdomen (tummy)

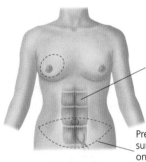

Transverse rectus abdominis muscle

Preoperative surgical markings on section to transfer

2. The flap is then attached to the chest wall to create the shape of a breast and connected to a new blood supply in the breast region

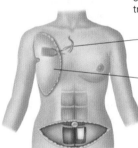

New blood supply

Flap is reattached at predetermined site

3. Final appearance with nipple reconstruction

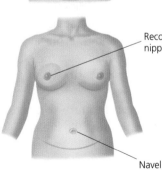

Reconstructed nipple

Navel repositioned

Generally the blood supply from a free flap is better than from a pedicled flap. This means that once the wounds have healed there are usually fewer long-term problems and fewer abdominal complications using a free flap.

However, the process of joining together the small blood vessels for a free flap is sometimes not straightforward and the risk of the whole flap dying is greater with this method.

One of the problems with taking muscle from the abdomen is that it weakens the abdominal wall. The surgeon will usually place a mesh to fill the gap where the muscle has been removed to try to stop the development of hernias or bulges. This is not always successful, however, and some people who have had this type of operation complain of some weakness of the muscle of the abdomen.

Other flaps

It is possible to reconstruct the breast using fat and skin from the lower abdomen over the rectus abdominis muscle without taking any muscle. The blood vessels are followed through the muscle but the muscle itself is not damaged. This operation takes much longer and is technically a much more difficult operation. The name of the blood vessels used are the **d**eep **i**nferior **ep**igastric vessels, so it is often called a DIEP flap for short.

It is possible to take skin and fat from the buttock area to reconstruct the breast. These are uncommon procedures in the UK, and are used only in patients who are unsuitable for other types of reconstruction.

Lumpectomy and immediate breast reconstruction

Large cancers are usually treated by mastectomy but it is sometime possible to remove large cancers by lumpectomy and then reconstruct the breast immediately with tissue from elsewhere in the body. The most common tissue used is muscle and skin from the back. Part of the latissimus dorsi muscle with some overlying fat is used. This is known as a latissimus dorsi mini-flap.

Placement of a mini-flap can be performed at the same time as removal of the cancer. Another option is to remove the cancer, check that all the cancer has been removed, and a few days later go back and fill the space in the breast by a mini-flap.

There are other flaps of tissue and muscle that are used in a few centres. The basis of these flaps is having a large enough blood vessel to supply the tissue to be moved, so that the flap survives after it is transferred to the breast. If you are suitable for one of these flaps your doctor will discuss this with you in detail.

Reconstruction of the breast in women who have had a lumpectomy and radiotherapy

Up to one in five women who have breast-conserving treatment finds that the treated breast is smaller than the other side. In this situation, it is possible to make the treated breast bigger or the opposite normal breast smaller. The results of this can be excellent.

Reducing both breasts at the time of lumpectomy

Some women who have cancer and have larger breasts may opt not only to have the cancer removed but at the same time to make both breasts smaller (therapeutic mammoplasty). The same approach that is used in breast reduction allows large volumes of breast tissue to be removed, allowing large areas of cancer or pre-cancer DCIS to be excised, and at the same time producing a satisfactory cosmetic outcome. This surgery is usually possible only in larger units and is ideally carried out by two surgeons working together, a breast surgeon and a plastic surgeon. The results are excellent and most patients are happy that their cancer is gone and their breasts are smaller and sit slightly higher than before surgery.

Surgery to the other breast

If you are having a breast reconstruction the surgeon carrying out your breast reconstruction will try to match the shape of the reconstructed breast with your remaining breast. This is not always possible so it may be suggested that you have an operation on your normal breast to change it so that it matches the reconstructed breast.

This may involve reducing the size of the other breast or lifting it to reduce its natural droop. This type of surgery does leave scars but any scars will fade with time and this may be the only way of getting a satisfactory match to the opposite breast.

Being realistic about breast reconstruction

Every effort is made to achieve the best possible result from reconstruction but not every person will achieve a perfect match to their opposite normal breast. When undressed you may find that your reconstructed breast has less of a droop than the opposite normal breast.

If the shape of your reconstructed breast differs greatly from the opposite breast it is possible to wear an external prosthesis over the reconstructed breast.

If you are unhappy with your reconstructed breast discuss this with your surgeon. If all your questions are not answered or you still feel unhappy, you can request a second opinion.

You can still have radiotherapy or chemotherapy if you have had a flap reconstruction. The only problem with radiotherapy is that, if you have an implant, it is more likely that you will develop some tightening around the implant than women who do not require this treatment.

This tightening is called capsular contracture and it occasionally happens even in women who do not have radiotherapy. When any foreign body, such as an implant, is put into your body, it reacts by forming fibrous tissue or a capsule around it.

Over a few months this fibrous tissue may contract and in some patients the contraction is quite marked, resulting in hardening and change in the shape of the implant that can be uncomfortable and spoil the shape of the reconstructed breast.

About five to ten per cent of women develop marked capsular contracture. This can be treated by removing the implant and taking away the capsule.

The same implant or a new one is then placed. This is usually successful at improving the shape and the capsule does not usually form for a second time.

Lipofilling

This is a new procedure, developed from liposuction techniques. It is used to fill in dents or defects in the breast, or to enlarge a breast. It involves taking fat from one part of the body, for example the inner part of the thigh or the abdomen, and then injecting it carefully into the breast. It may be done in two or three stages and can be done using a local anaesthetic, but usually requires a general anaesthetic.

Nipple reconstruction

It is usually but not always necessary to remove the nipple during mastectomy but it is possible to reconstruct a nipple later. This is generally performed a few months after breast reconstruction so that the nipple that is reconstructed can be matched in its shape and position to the other nipple.

In patients having both breasts removed it is often possible to save one nipple and this can be split into two and grafted on to produce two small nipples during the first reconstruction operation.

A reconstructed nipple is usually created from skin on the reconstructed breast. Having made the nipple it will take six to eight weeks to heal and settle down, and then the area is suitable for tattooing to produce a correct colour match to the other nipple. Tattooing is usually painless and can give a very realistic appearance to the nipple and the surrounding area called the areola.

It is important to be realistic about a reconstructed nipple. It will not behave in the same way as the opposite nipple and will not have any sensation.

It is quite difficult to reconstruct very large nipples so if you do have a large nipple on the other breast, one option is to take part of the normal nipple and transfer it across to reconstruct the new nipple; this is called nipple sharing.

Nipple prostheses

Another option is to wear a stick-on nipple. These are readily available from your breast care nurse.

Nipple reconstruction – nipple flap

Skin on the new breast can be folded into a nipple shape – this is called a nipple flap. There are different techniques and the procedure is usually done under a local anaesthetic and you should be able to go home the same day.

Tattooing after breast reconstruction can give the reconstructed nipple a very good appearance.

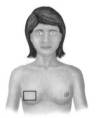

Location

Batwing
1. The outline is marked on the skin

2. The three arms of the star are cut out

3. Two lateral arms are folded over from the base and sutured together to form a cylindrical mound. The surrounding base skin is sutured together

4. The central arm provides the top section. This creates a projecting structure that is self-supporting and stable

It is possible to make a nipple specifically for you. A mould is taken of your other nipple, which allows the stick-on nipple to be a very close match to the shape and colour of your other nipple.

KEY POINTS

■ In most women it is possible to reconstruct a breast shape after mastectomy

■ This can be done either at the time of mastectomy or later

■ Breast reconstruction uses breast implants and/or skin and muscle flaps to bring tissue from elsewhere in the body

■ Breast reconstruction can be a major undertaking for you and it is important to be realistic about your expectations

■ In women with cancer who have larger breasts, the cancer can be removed and both breasts made smaller – a procedure called therapeutic mammoplasty

Emotional response to the diagnosis of breast cancer

How can a diagnosis affect you?

Any breast problem, even one that is minor in health terms, is likely to affect a woman psychologically and emotionally as well as physically. Very many women are sensitive about the shape and size of their breasts and breasts are an important aspect of any woman's sexuality. A woman may be concerned about her partner's likely reaction to any breast problem, as well as her own.

From your perspective, anything being wrong with your breasts may have a damaging effect on your self-image and so take on an importance way beyond its significance in pure health terms. Of course, no two women will react in exactly the same way and your reaction to any breast problem is unique, but knowing that these kinds of worries are normal may help to keep them in proportion.

Talking it over and getting support
Support from medical staff

Doctors and nurses who treat women regularly and manage a full range of breast problems are well aware of the psychological aspects of breast disease. Usually, they will ask about your emotional reactions and whether you have any worries that you would like to talk over and it really is worthwhile if asked to take the opportunity to raise anything that's on your mind.

Some people find this difficult, perhaps feeling that nothing can be done to help or that they would be wasting the doctor's or nurse's time. This is very much not the case, and keeping your concerns to yourself is likely to do more harm than good in the long run. You should be offered support and advice by the doctors and nurses involved in your care.

Other sources of support

There are numerous support groups that can offer more for those who want it. In particular, there is a lot of help available for women who have breast cancer as well as for their families.

You should be offered the opportunity to meet and talk to others in a similar situation. This is usually someone who has had breast cancer treated successfully and has some training in helping other people cope. Breast Cancer Care offer this service and contact details are on page 221.

When it is a member of your family or close friend who has a serious condition such as breast cancer, it can be hard to express your worries and to seek emotional support for yourself.

It's easy to believe that you shouldn't compete with the patient's needs for help even though you will have your own concerns and worries. Many of the self-help groups provide support for people in this situation.

KEY POINTS

- Breast conditions can often affect women psychologically and emotionally

- Do not keep your concerns to yourself but share them with your carers

- Support should be available from your doctors and nurses, and is also available from self-help groups

Follow-up after breast cancer treatment

Follow-up checks

There are three main reasons for patients being seen in hospital for follow-up after treatment of breast cancer:

1 To detect a cancer that returns or a new breast cancer that develops as early as possible

2 To detect and treat side effects and problems that occur as a result of treatment

3 To give psychological support

To detect a cancer that returns or a new breast cancer that develops as early as possible

As we have stressed earlier in the book early detection is paramount in effecting a successful treatment.

The chances of cancer returning in most women are, however, extremely small. The best way of detecting further disease in the breasts is by having regular follow-up mammograms. Most women do not require regular follow-up clinical examination or regular clinic visits as most recurrences are found on the mammograms or by the patients themselves.

To detect and treat side effects and problems that occur as a result of treatment

This includes side effects of drugs but also problems related to your surgery such as mismatch between the two breasts after breast-conserving surgery or problems with your scar after mastectomy.

The most common of these is extra tissue at the ends of the mastectomy scar, particularly at the end of the scar under the arm. These extra portions of tissue are known as 'dog's ears' and can be trimmed at a second operation to leave a flatter and more comfortable scar.

Other problems after surgery include a swollen arm (lymphoedema) which develops in 1 in 20 of those who have all the lymph nodes removed.

To give psychological support

Psychological support is necessary because it is very common for women to be anxious or depressed the first few years after a diagnosis of breast cancer.

Breast care nurses play an important role in supporting patients during treatment and after treatment finishes. You should have contact details of your breast care nurse and you should phone them if you experience any problems, physical or psychological.

Continuing support

The chances of the cancer returning are now lower

than they have ever been. Although you will have regular visits for the first two years to have an examination by a doctor or nurse, the chances of them finding anything wrong is very small. After the first one to two years you will get regular mammograms but do not need a clinic visit.

It is important that you remain alert to problems and report anything abnormal that you feel to your doctors or nurses as soon as you discover a problem. Each year a mammogram will be organised – which is the best way of detecting new problems at an early stage.

You will not have regular X-rays or scans to look for cancer elsewhere in the body because this is not worthwhile. The major reason is that the chances of finding disease are very small, so the tests are unnecessary.

At any hospital appointment you should report all problems that you are experiencing, including all the side effects of any drugs that you are taking.

You will be asked how you are feeling and coping. It is important to be honest and let the doctors or nurses know of any anxieties or worries. You may be given a questionnaire to complete to assess how you are feeling and what effect the breast cancer is having on your life.

You should have regular mammograms for the rest of your life even if you do not attend a breast clinic. Discuss with your doctors or nurses how you can ensure that this is organised and where you should attend.

Hormone treatments for breast cancer may continue for up to 10 years. If you are on prolonged treatment you will need regular scans of your bone density to check that you do not develop osteoporosis (thinning of the bones). Your hospital doctor, specialist nurse or GP will organise this.

Glossary

Here is a list of terms that are used throughout the book or that you may hear during your treatment:

Adenocarcinoma: a cancer that develops in a gland forming tissue similar to that in the breast. This term is not in general use but it may appear on your pathology report.

Adjuvant systemic therapy: treatment given after surgery and/or radiotherapy to reduce the chance of cancer returning; includes treatments such as chemotherapy or hormonal therapy that affect the whole body.

Advanced breast cancer: cancer that has spread (metastasised) to other parts of the body through the bloodstream.

Amenorrhoea: absence or stoppage of menstrual periods.

Anorexia: loss of appetite.

Anthracyclines: group of chemotherapy drugs including doxorubicin (Adriamycin) and epirubicin.

These are the most commonly used drugs in breast cancer. Mitozantrone is another type of anthracycline that is used occasionally to treat breast cancer.

Anti-inflammatory drugs: these are used to treat breast and bone pain or areas of inflammation and include paracetamol and ibuprofen.

Areola: the pigmented area of skin around the nipple.

Aromatase: the enzyme that converts male hormones to oestrogen.

Aromatase inhibitors: drugs that block the aromatase enzyme and stop the production of oestrogen. Effective only in postmenopausal women.

Aspiration: removal of fluid or cells from a collection of fluid such as a cyst or a breast lump.

Asymmetry: difference in appearance of two sides of the body, usually used when comparing the two breasts.

Atypical hyperplasia: abnormal cells within the breast lobule that have increased in number and expand the lobule but do not fill all the spaces in the lobule; part of what is now called lobular neoplasia.

Axilla: the armpit.

Axillary clearance: removal of all lymph nodes from underneath the axilla.

Axillary dissection: removal of some or all the lymph glands from under the armpit.

Axillary nodes: lymph glands in the armpit that drain the lymph from the breast.

Axillary sampling: removal of a few lymph glands, usually four, from the armpit.

Benign: not cancerous.

Bilateral: both sides of the body.

Bilateral prophylactic mastectomy: surgical removal of both breasts to reduce the risk of development of breast cancer.

Biopsy: removal of a sample of tissue which is then examined under the microscope to check cause of a lump.

Bone scan: test to check for cancer in the bones.

***BRCA*-1 gene**: the first gene to be identified which is associated with breast cancer in some families; abnormalities in this gene are linked to breast cancer in certain families. Women with an abnormal *BRCA*-1 gene are also at increased risk of ovarian cancer.

***BRCA*-2 gene**: the second gene abnormalities in this gene have been linked to breast cancer in certain families. There is also an increased risk of ovarian cancer in women with an abnormal *BRCA*-2 gene. Men with abnormal *BRCA*-2 genes may also develop breast cancer.

Breast-conserving surgery: an operation that removes the cancer and some surrounding normal tissue with the intention of maintaining the breast shape.

Breast reconstruction: an operation to rebuild the breast to match the other side.

Calcification: small calcium deposits in the breast that can be seen on a mammogram.

Cancer: a growth of abnormal tissue, the growth of which is uncontrolled. Cancer cells invade surrounding tissues and can also spread through the bloodstream and lymphatic system to other parts of the body.

Capsule: the fibrous tissue that forms around foreign material such as an implant.

Capsular contraction: contraction of the fibrous capsule that develops around an implant, which can cause the implant to feel hard and alter in shape.

Cellulitis: infection of the skin or tissues under the skin of the breast.

Chemotherapy: treatment with drugs aimed at destroying cancer cells.

Clear margin: a rim of normal tissue around a cancer that is essential when performing breast-conserving surgery.

Clinical oncologist: a doctor who specialises in treatment of cancer with radiotherapy. Some clinical oncologists also give chemotherapy.

Clinical trial: research studies that involve patients. These studies are designed to find better ways to prevent, detect or treat cancer.

Combination chemotherapy: a combination of drugs as compared with a single drug chemotherapy.

Contralateral tumour: a cancer in the opposite breast to the one affected by breast cancer.

Core biopsy: removal of a thin sliver of tissue from the breast using a needle.

CT: computed tomography – a type of X-ray where a computer is used to produce detailed pictures. It is particularly useful for looking at the liver, bone and brain, to tell whether cancer is present.

Cyst: a collection of fluid within the breast usually seen around the menopause.

Cytology: examination of cells removed with a needle from a breast lump under the microscope. This requires an expert pathologist or cytologist.

Diagnostic radiographer: a person trained in the taking of X-ray pictures. A therapeutic radiographer is one who is involved in giving radiotherapy.

DIEP flap: **d**eep **i**nferior **ep**igastric artery **p**erforator flap used for breast reconstruction.

DNA: deoxyribonucleic acid – the material that contains the genetic code.

Drain: a tube placed at the end of an operation to remove any fluids that collect under the wound.

Ducts: hollow tubes that either connect the breast lobule to the nipple or take fluid from one part of the body to another, such as from the breast to the lymph nodes.

Ductal carcinoma *in situ* (DCIS): non-invasive cancer arising in the terminal duct lobular unit of the breast.

Endocrine therapy: drugs that interfere with hormones and are used to treat the breast cancer.

Expander: an inflatable implant.

Flap: a portion of tissue that is moved from one part of the body to another.

Free flap: a flap that is detached from one part of the body and moved to another part where the blood vessels are reconnected.

Gene: sequence of DNA required to make a particular protein.

Grade: describes how closely a cancer resembles normal tissue of the same type and also reflects the cancer's rate of growth. Low-grade or grade 1 cancers closely resemble normal tissue whereas grade 3 cancers least resemble normal tissue and grow faster.

Gynaecomastia: male breast enlargement.

Haematoma: collection of blood beneath the skin.

Haemorrhage: bleeding.

HER2: there are four human epidermal growth factor receptors. This was the second to be described and in 15 to 20 per cent of cancer there is more HER2 protein on the surface on the cell than in normal breast cells and this causes the cell to grow faster. This HER2 protein can be targeted by the drug trastuzumab (Herceptin).

Herceptin: a drug also known as trastuzumab that is effective against cancers that are HER2 (human epidermal growth factor receptor 2) positive.

Hodgkin's disease: a type of cancer that involves the lymph nodes.

Hormone: a chemical substance produced by glands that enters the bloodstream and affects other organs.

Hormone receptor test: a test to measure the amount of proteins known as hormone receptors in breast cancer tissue. A high level of hormone receptors means that hormones are important to help the cancer grow and therefore removal or blockage of the hormones is likely to be effective at stopping the cancer growing.

Hormone replacement therapy (HRT): drugs that usually contain oestrogen with or without a progesterone-like substance, which are used to treat the symptoms of the menopause.

Hormone treatment: treatment of cancer by removing, blocking or adding hormones.

Hyperplasia: an increase in the number of normal cells in a tissue.

Hysterectomy: an operation in which the uterus (womb) and cervix are removed.

Imaging: tests such as X-rays or ultrasound used to produce pictures of certain areas of the body.

Implant: used for breast reconstruction, usually filled with silicone gel and occasionally with saline.

Infertility: inability to produce children.

Infiltrating cancer: cancer that invades surrounding tissue.

Inflammatory breast cancer: a rare type of breast cancer in which the cancer cells block the lymph channels in the skin under the breast. The breast is characteristically swollen, red and warm, and the skin of the breast may appear pitted and have ridges. It produces an orange peel-like appearance – skin thickening – peau d'orange.

In situ: these cancers do not invade beyond the tissue in which they arise so a ductal carcinoma *in situ* is limited within the terminal duct lobular unit and draining ducts.

Internal mammary nodes: nodes behind the edge of the breastbone.

Intraductal: within a duct.

Intraductal cancer: this is the same as DCIS, that is non-invasive cancer in the ducts and lobule.

Intravenous: injection into a vein.

Invasive cancer: invasive cancers have the ability to spread beyond the lobules and ducts in which they formed into the surrounding breast tissue. They can also spread to other parts of the body.

Latissimus dorsi muscle: a large broad muscle just under the skin of the upper back.

LHRH agonist: a drug that mimics luteinising hormone-releasing hormone (LHRH) and results in reduction of production of oestrogen from the ovary.

Lobular carcinoma *in situ* (LCIS): abnormal cells that fill and expand the terminal duct lobular unit. These are round cells and LCIS looks different under the microscope from DCIS.

Lobular neoplasia: a term for the two conditions previously known as lobular carcinoma *in* situ *and* atypical lobular hyperplasia.

Local: affecting the breast and chest wall.

Local therapy: treatment that is directed to the cancer in the breast and the area close to it.

Locally advanced breast cancer: a cancer that is large and involves the skin or muscles of the chest wall but has not necessarily spread elsewhere.

Lumpectomy: removal of the cancer with a rim of normal tissue.

Lymph: the colourless fluid that leaks out of blood and then travels back through the lymphatic system to lymph nodes. It can carry cells from cancers to the lymph glands.

Lymph nodes: small and bean shaped, these are located along the channels of the lymphatic system. Lymph nodes store special cells that fight off bacteria. They can be affected by cancer cells. Clusters of lymph glands are found under the arm, under the breastbone and in the groin, neck, chest and abdomen.

Lymphoedema: a condition in which excess fluid builds up in tissues and causes swelling. This can affect both the arms and the legs.

Lymphovascular invasion: cancer cells that have spread into lymph channels or blood vessels.

Magnetic resonance imaging (MRI): uses strong magnets linked to a computer to create detailed pictures of areas inside the body.

Malignant: a tumour that is able to spread to other parts of the body.

Mammography: use of X-rays to create a picture of the breast.

Mastectomy: surgical removal of the whole breast.

Mastopexy: surgical uplift of the breast.

Medical oncologist: a doctor who specialises in treatment of cancers with drugs.

Menarche: age at which a woman's periods begin.

Menopause: the change of life (climacteric), the time when a woman's periods stop.

Menstrual cycle: the hormonal changes that take place every month.

Metastasis: spread of cancer to other parts of the body. Breast cancers commonly spread or metastasise to the lungs, liver, bone or brain.

Microcalcification: a tiny deposit of calcium in the breast that cannot be felt but is detected by a mammogram. A cluster of microcalcification may indicate that a cancer is present.

Micrometastasis: very small group of cancer cells that have spread to another part of the body such as the lymph node.

Multicentric tumour: more than one area of tumour in the same breast but widely apart.

Multidisciplinary care: management by a team of doctors usually involving a surgeon, oncologists, radiologists and pathologists.

Multifocal disease: disease affecting more than one area in the breast but close together.

Multimodality treatment: use of a combination of different types of treatment for breast cancer, usually a combination of surgery, radiotherapy and drug therapy.

Neoadjuvant therapy: drug treatments that are given before surgery.

Neoplasm: abnormal growth of tissue; can be benign or malignant.

Oncologist: a doctor who specialises in treating cancer. Some oncologists specialise in a particular type of cancer treatment – for example, a medical or a clinical oncologist.

Oncology: study of cancers.

Oncoplastic technique: surgical technique combining the specialities of cancer surgery to excise the cancer (onco-) and plastic surgery to reconstruct after removal of the cancer (plastic).

Osteoporosis: softening of the bones and bone loss that occur with increasing age or secondary to drug treatment that lowers the oestrogen level in the body.

Ovarian suppression or ablation: suppression of oestrogen production from the ovaries or surgical removal of the ovaries.

p53: a gene involved in controlling the growth of cells. An abnormal *p53* gene can result in development of multiple cancers including breast cancer. This occurs as part of a rare syndrome known as the Li–Fraumeni syndrome.

Palliation: the activity of relieving a symptom without affecting the cause.

Palliative treatment: treatment that does not alter the course of the disease but improves the quality of life.

Pathologist: a doctor who specialises in diagnosis of disease using a microscope.

Pedicled flap: a flap of tissue, usually skin, muscle and fat, that is left attached to its blood supply and is moved to another part of the body. Pedicled flaps are a common method of breast reconstruction.

Port of an expander/implant: a reservoir that is attached to an expander. It allows the injection of saline into the expander.

Postmenopausal: after the menopause.

Pre-cancerous: a term used to describe a condition that occurs before cancer develops.

Progesterone: one of the two female hormones; the other is oestrogen.

Prognosis: the probable outcome of the course of disease.

Prosthesis: artificial replacement for a body part.

Radioactive: giving off radiation.

Radiologist: a doctor who specialises in imaging and interpreting images of areas inside the body. The images are produced by X-rays, sound waves or other types of energy such as magnetism.

Radiotherapy: treatment with high-energy X-rays to kill cancer cells.

Recurrence: a cancer that returns or re-grows either in the area around the site of initial surgery (local recurrence) or somewhere else in the body (systemic recurrence).

Relapse: the return of signs and symptoms of disease after apparently successful treatment.

Remission: successful treatment and control of a disease.

Risk factors: something that increases the chances of developing a disease.

Screening: identifying disease at a stage before it has caused symptoms.

Sentinel lymph node biopsy: removal of one or more nodes that are the first nodes that drain a particular organ such as the breast.

Sentinel node of the breast: the first node receiving lymphatic drainage from the breast. This is usually in the lower part of the armpit. There is rarely one sentinel node. The average is three.

Seroma: collection of fluid underneath the skin.

Side effects: undesirable effects of treatment.

Silicone: synthetic material used to fill breast implants.

Stage: the extent of cancer spread in the body.

Staging: performing tests and examinations to determine the extent of cancer spread.

Stereotactic guidance: using two X-rays from different angles to pinpoint the exact location of a lesion in the breast that cannot be felt to allow a biopsy to be performed. Stereotactic guidance is also used to place a 'wire' in the breast to guide the surgeon when excising an area of calcifications or other abnormality.

Supraclavicular: the area above the collarbone. This usually refers to lymph glands in this area.

Systemic therapy: treatment that uses drugs that travel through the bloodstream to reach all cells throughout the body.

Tamoxifen: a drug that blocks the oestrogen receptors found on the surface of normal and cancerous cells in the breast.

Terminal duct lobular unit: the milk-producing part of the breast where cancer starts.

TRAM flap: **t**ransverse **r**ectus **a**bdominis **m**yocutaneous flap – a flap of tissue taken from the patient's lower abdomen that includes muscle.

Ultrasonography: ultrasound is a test that uses sound waves. These are bounced off tissues and the echoes are converted into a picture.

Wide excision: surgical removal of a lump with a margin of normal tissue surrounding the tumour.

X-ray: high-energy radiation used in low doses to diagnose disease and in high doses to treat cancer.

Further information

If you would like to talk to someone else who has been through similar experiences, trained volunteers can be contacted through Breast Cancer Care (see below) or local self-help groups. The following national associations provide emotional support and practical help to women with breast cancer or to their friends and relatives.

Useful addresses

We have included the following organisations because, on preliminary investigation, they may be of use to the reader. However, we do not have first-hand experience of each organisation and so cannot guarantee the organisation's integrity. The reader must therefore exercise his or her own discretion and judgement when making further enquiries.

Breakthrough Breast Cancer

Weston House, 3rd Floor, 246 High Holborn
London WC1V 7EX

Tel: 020 7025 2400
Freephone info line: 0808 010 0200
Website: www.breakthrough.org.uk

A charity with aims to raise awareness of breast cancer issues among the public and to campaign hard to keep breast cancer high on the media and political agendas. Has established a research centre for breast cancer research and treatment.

Breast Cancer Care
5–13 Great Suffolk Street
London SE1 0NS
Freephone: 0808 800 6000 (Mon–Fri 9am–5pm, Sat 9am–2pm)
Textphone: 0808 800 6001
Website: www.breastcancercare.org.uk

Specialist breast care nurses provide practical advice, medical information and support to women concerned about breast cancer. Volunteers who have had breast cancer themselves assist in giving emotional support to cancer patients and their partners. Free leaflets and a prosthesis-fitting service also provided.

Breast Cancer Care Scotland and Northern Ireland
169 Elderslie Street
Glasgow G3 7JR
Tel: 0845 077 1892

Specialist breast care nurses provide practical advice, medical information and support to women concerned about breast cancer. Volunteers who have had breast cancer themselves assist in giving emotional support to cancer patients and their partners. Free leaflets and a prosthesis-fitting service also provided.

Breast Cancer Haven
Effie Road
London SW6 1TB
Tel: 020 7384 0099
Website: www.breastcancerhaven.org.uk

A charity providing support centres for women with breast cancer. Provides complementary and alternative medicine to help heal the mind, body and spirit through group support and individual therapy programmes. Works with health-care professionals to promote integrated breast cancer care. Centres in London, Hereford and Leeds.

British Association for Counselling and Psychotherapy
15 St John's Business Park
Lutterworth LE17 4HB
Tel: 01455 883300
Website: www.counselling.co.uk

Registered charity working towards the promotion and regulation of counselling and psychotherapy, both for the profession and the public's benefit.

Cancer Research UK
PO Box 123, Lincoln's Inn Fields
London WC2A 3PX
Tel: 020 7121 6699 (customer services)
Tel: 020 7242 0200 (switchboard)

Tel: 0808 800 4040 (information nurses)
Website: www.cancerresearchuk.org

Funds research into cancer and education. It provides
information to people with cancer and their carers.

CancerHelp UK

Cancer Information Department, Cancer Research UK,
PO Box 123, Lincoln's Inn Fields
London WC2A 3PX
Freephone: 0808 800 4040 (Mon–Fri 9am–5pm)
Website: www.cancerhelp.org.uk

A free information service about cancer and cancer
care for people with cancer and their families. Brought
to you by Cancer Research UK (see above). Believes
that information about cancer should be freely
available to all and written in a way that people can
easily understand.

Carers UK

20 Great Dover Street
London SE1 4LX
Tel: 020 7378 4999
Carers' line: 0808 808 7777 (Wed, Thurs 10am–12
noon, 2–4pm)
Website: www.carersuk.org

Offers information and support to all people who are
unpaid carers, looking after others with medical or
other problems.

Crossroads Caring for Carers
10 Regent Place
Rugby, Warwickshire CV21 2PN
Helpline: 0845 450 0350
Website: www.crossroads.org.uk

Supports and delivers high-quality services for carers
and people with care needs via its local branches.

The Daisy Network
PO Box 183
Rossendale BB4 6WZ
Website: www.daisynetwork.org.uk

A premature menopause support group.

Hereditary Breast Cancer Helpline
Information Centre, St Anne Cottage, Over Haddon
Derby DE45
Tel: 01629 81300

Macmillan Cancer Relief (now merged with Cancerbackup)
89 Albert Embankment
London SE1 7UQ
Tel: 020 7840 7840
Freephone: 0800 808 0000
Website: www.macmillan.org.uk

A national charity dedicated to improving the quality of
life for people with cancer and their families. Funds
Macmillan Nursing Services for home care, hospital and
hospice support. Financial help also given. Incorporates
Cancerlink, which provides training and consultancy

for the many self-help and support groups and organisations nationwide. Advises people setting up new groups; these are listed in a free and annually updated directory. Through merger with Cancerbackup, provides a very wide range of free publications available on a large number of different cancers, treatments and related issues.

Maggie's Centres
Maggie's Centre Edinburgh, The Stables, Western General Hospital, Crewe Road
Edinburgh EH4 2XU
Tel: 0131 537 2456
Website: www.maggiescentres.org

Founded in Edinburgh by a patient called Maggie Keswick Jenks who felt that there needed to be centres close to cancer hospitals where patients and relatives could go; these should be run especially for and by patients. Also provide valuable sources of information as well as support. Provide internet access in all their locations. The charity aims to help all people with cancer to be healthy in mind and body. There are centres throughout the country with plans to open further centres.

Marie Curie Cancer Care
89 Albert Embankment
London SE1 7TP
Tel: 020 7599 7777
Website: www.mariecurie.org.uk

A national charity that runs ten specialist palliative care hospices around the UK. Provides a national palliative care nursing service in the home. Involved in research and in the education of health-care professionals in a range of cancer and palliative care programmes.

National Association of Citizens Advice Bureau

Myddleton House, 115–123 Pentonville Road
London N1 9LZ
Tel: 020 7833 2181

Look in the local telephone directory or library for the address of the nearest Citizens Advice Bureau. There are 2,800 bureaux nationwide and all of these can provide free, impartial, confidential advice and help. Most specialist units have access to support funds and can help people who want to apply.

Tenovus Cancer Information Centre

9th Floor, Gleider House, Ty Glas Road, Llanishen
Cardiff CF14 5BD
Tel: 029 2076 8850
Website: www.tenovus.org.uk

Making a difference to people with cancer and their families by delivering cancer treatment and support in their local communities.

Ulster Cancer Foundation

40–44 Eglantine Avenue
Belfast, Northern Ireland BT9 6DX
Tel: 0800 783 3339
Website: www.ulstercancer.org

Activities supporting the vision of the day when cancer

is no longer a life-threatening disease – from funding research into new and better treatments for cancer, undertaking education programmes to helping people reduce their risk of developing cancer.

Other useful addresses
Benefits Enquiry Line
Freephone: 0800 882200 (8.30am–6.30pm weekdays)
Textphone: 0800 243355
Website: www.dwp.gov.uk
N. Ireland: 0800 220674

Government agency giving information and advice on sickness and disability benefits for people with disabilities and their carers.

National Cancer Institute
NCI Public Inquiries Office, Room 3036A, 6116 Executive Boulevard
Bethesda, MD 20892-8322, USA
Tel: + 1 800 422 6237 (Mon–Fri 09.00am–4.30pm local time)
Website: www.cancer.gov

American organisation funded by the government that provides cancer-related health information and funding for scientific research throughout the USA. Offers consumer-oriented information on a wide range of topics as well as descriptions of its research programmes for the general public and health professionals. Scientists will find detailed information on specific areas of research and funding opportunities.

National Institute for Health and Clinical Excellence (NICE)

MidCity Place, 71 High Holborn
London WC1V 6NA
Tel: 0845 003 7780
Website: www.nice.org.uk

Provides guidance on treatments and care for people using the NHS in England and Wales. Patient information leaflets are available for each piece of guidance issued.

NHS Direct

Tel: 0845 4647 (24 hours, 365 days a year)
Website: www.nhsdirect.nhs.uk

Offers confidential health-care advice, information and referral service. A good first port of call for any health advice.

NHS Smoking Helpline

Freephone: 0800 022 4332 (7am–11pm, 365 days a year)
Website: http://mokefree.nhs.uk
Pregnancy smoking helpline: 0800 169 9169 (12 noon–9pm, 365 days a year)

Have advice, help and encouragement on giving up smoking. Specialist advisers available to offer ongoing support to those who genuinely are trying to give up smoking. Can refer to local branches.

Patients' Association

PO Box 935
Harrow HA1 3YJ
Tel: 020 8423 9111

Helpline: 0845 608 4455
Website: www.patients-association.com

Provides advice on patients' rights, leaflets and
directory of self-help groups.

Quit (Smoking Quitlines)
63 St Mary's Axe
London EC3 8AA
Helpline: 0800 002200 (9am–9pm, 365 days a year)
Tel: 020 7469 0400
Website: www.quit.org.uk

Offers individual advice on giving up smoking in
English and Asian languages. Talks to schools on
smoking and pregnancy and can refer to local support
groups. Runs training courses for professionals.

Useful websites
BBC
www.bbc.co.uk/health
A helpful website: easy to navigate and offers lots of
useful advice and information. Also contains links to
other related topics.

Patient UK
www.patient.co.uk
Patient care website.

mikedixon.org.uk
A website that acts as a portal to allow access to the
websites listed above and provides sites of information
endorsed by Professor Mike Dixon, one of the authors.

Tak Tent Cancer Support – Scotland
www.taktent.org.uk

The internet as a further source of information

After reading this book, you may feel that you would like further information on the subject. The internet is of course an excellent place to look and there are many websites with useful information about medical disorders, related charities and support groups.

For those who do not have a computer at home some bars and cafes offer facilities for accessing the internet. These are listed in the Yellow Pages under 'Internet Bars and Cafes' and 'Internet Providers'. Your local library offers a similar facility and has staff to help you find the information that you need.

It should always be remembered, however, that the internet is unregulated and anyone is free to set up a website and add information to it. Many websites offer impartial advice and information that has been compiled and checked by qualified medical professionals. Some, on the other hand, are run by commercial organisations with the purpose of promoting their own products. Others still are run by pressure groups, some of which will provide carefully assessed and accurate information whereas others may be suggesting medications or treatments that are not supported by the medical and scientific community.

Unless you know the address of the website you want to visit – for example, www.familydoctor.co.uk – you may find the following guidelines useful when searching the internet for information.

Search engines and other searchable sites

Google (www.google.co.uk) is the most popular search engine used in the UK, followed by Yahoo! (http://uk.yahoo.com) and MSN (www.msn.co.uk). Also popular are the search engines provided by Internet Service Providers such as Tiscali and other sites such as the BBC site (www.bbc.co.uk).

In addition to the search engines that index the whole web, there are also medical sites with search facilities, which act almost like mini-search engines, but cover only medical topics or even a particular area of medicine. Again, it is wise to look at who is responsible for compiling the information offered to ensure that it is impartial and medically accurate. The NHS Direct site (www.nhsdirect.nhs.uk) is an example of a searchable medical site.

Links to many British medical charities can be found at the Association of Medical Research Charities website (www.amrc.org.uk) and at Charity Choice (www.charitychoice.co.uk).

Search phrases

Be specific when entering a search phrase. Searching for information on 'cancer' will return results for many different types of cancer as well as on cancer in general. You may even find sites offering astrological information. More useful results will be returned by using search phrases such as 'breast cancer' and 'treatments for breast cancer'. Both Google and Yahoo! offer an advanced search option that includes the ability to search for the exact phrase, enclosing the search phrase in quotes, that is, 'treatments for breast cancer' will have the same effect. Limiting a search to an exact phrase reduces the number of results returned but it is best to refine a search to an exact match only if you are not getting useful results with a normal search. Adding 'UK' to your search term will bring up mainly British sites, so a good phrase might be 'lung cancer' UK (don't include UK within the quotes).

Always remember the internet is international and unregulated. It holds a wealth of valuable information but individual sites may be biased, out of date or just plain wrong. Family Doctor Publications accepts no responsibility for the content of links published in this series.

Be wary of any special clinics offering treatment not available on the NHS. Some charge exorbitant fees for treatments for which there is no proven benefit. Some sites offer dietary advice, but again be wary. The evidence shows that women who have a balanced diet together with regular exercise have the best survival. Fad diets such as avoiding dairy products are of no proven value and may do harm. Local websites provide details of exercise or walking groups. The value of regular exercise after a diagnosis of breast cancer is well recognised in terms of improving both well-being and long-term survival.

Index

Your pages

We have included the following pages because they may help you manage your illness or condition and its treatment.

Before an appointment with a health professional, it can be useful to write down a short list of questions of things that you do not understand, so that you can make sure that you do not forget anything.

Some of the sections may not be relevant to your circumstances.

We are always pleased to receive constructive criticism or suggestions about how to improve the books. You can contact us at:

Email: familydoctor@btinternet.com
Letter: Family Doctor Publications
          PO Box 4664
          Poole
          BH15 1NN

Thank you

Health-care contact details

Name:

Job title:

Place of work:

Tel:

Name:

Job title:

Place of work:

Tel:

Name:

Job title:

Place of work:

Tel:

Name:

Job title:

Place of work:

Tel:

Significant past health events – illnesses/ operations/investigations/treatments

Event	Month	Year	Age (at time)

Appointments for health care

Name:

Place:

Date:

Time:

Tel:

Name:

Place:

Date:

Time:

Tel:

Name:

Place:

Date:

Time:

Tel:

Name:

Place:

Date:

Time:

Tel:

Appointments for health care

Name:

Place:

Date:

Time:

Tel:

Name:

Place:

Date:

Time:

Tel:

Name:

Place:

Date:

Time:

Tel:

Name:

Place:

Date:

Time:

Tel:

Current medication(s) prescribed by your doctor

Medicine name:

Purpose:

Frequency & dose:

Start date:

End date:

Medicine name:

Purpose:

Frequency & dose:

Start date:

End date:

Medicine name:

Purpose:

Frequency & dose:

Start date:

End date:

Medicine name:

Purpose:

Frequency & dose:

Start date:

End date:

Other medicines/supplements you are taking, not prescribed by your doctor

Medicine/treatment:

Purpose:

Frequency & dose:

Start date:

End date:

Medicine/treatment:

Purpose:

Frequency & dose:

Start date:

End date:

Medicine/treatment:

Purpose:

Frequency & dose:

Start date:

End date:

Medicine/treatment:

Purpose:

Frequency & dose:

Start date:

End date:

Questions to ask at appointments
(Note: do bear in mind that doctors work under great time
pressure, so long lists may not be helpful for either of you)

_____

_____

_____

_____

_____

_____

_____

_____

_____

_____

_____

_____

_____

_____

_____

_____

_____

_____

_____

_____

_____

_____

Questions to ask at appointments
(Note: do bear in mind that doctors work under great time
pressure, so long lists may not be helpful for either of you)

Notes

_____

_____

_____

_____

_____

_____

_____

_____

_____

_____

_____

_____

_____

_____

_____

_____

_____

_____

_____

_____

_____

_____

_____

_____

_____

Notes

Notes